For Rachel, who gave me the love
I needed to be able to write this book.

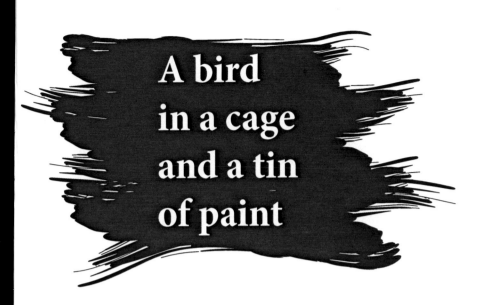

A bird
in a cage
and a tin
of paint

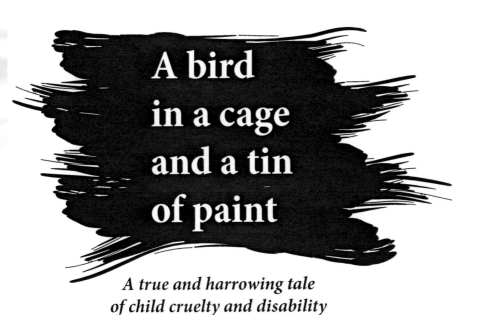

A bird in a cage and a tin of paint

A true and harrowing tale
of child cruelty and disability

Chris Stewart

THIS BOOK IS A PUBLICATION OF
McQueen Publishing
4 Johnson Close
Lancaster
LA1 5EU

ISBN 978 0 9573374 1 1

Printed by Berforts Information Press
in the United Kingdom

Contents

Chapter

1   Beginning the Realisation
2   A Traumatic Birth
3   The Horse and Harrison's Dairy
4   Stonegate Drive
5   The Knife Attack
6   My Brother Alan and I
7   A Tin of Paint and a Cartoon House
8   Taking my 'Pets' Around
9   Early Holidays with Dad
10   My Troubles in the Infants
11   My Frist Love
12   Ringing the Bell
13   My Little Friends
14   Winter and the Grey Snow Falling
15   Dad Chucked Out
16   The Weybridge Holiday
17   Hospital Visit Number 1
18   Punishment in the Winter Elements
19   Whit Walks and Summer Days

Contents

Chapter

20   Winter and Those 'Thank you' letters

21   Contact With Dad and His Side of the Family

22   The Secret Smokers

23   Church

24   The Juniors - Knobley and Dunce

25   Piano Lessons and Being Late for the Blackley Visit

26   Dr Smith and a Claim to Fame

27   Mother Leaving Us

28   Living with Aunty Julian in Denton

29   Swinton Baths

30   The Canyon in Wardley Woods

31   Burning the Field

32   My Sister Margaret and Our Code

33   Rape!

34   Mrs Bleasant

35   My Swan Song at Moorside School

36   That Damned Eleven Plus Exam

37   Beth Moulam

Foreword

Dear reader,

The following story is a true and my best recollection, of the life I had as a child. It may be slightly tinted with time. The tales told to me about my birth by the aunts there at the time when I was too young to remember may influence it. It may have the sting of my tears distorting some of the facts as I saw through those tears in times of trauma.

My story starts in Liverpool, on an art therapy course at the Tate gallery. Liverpool was alien to my childhood but I now recognise the need to go to some other, neutral place to view the happenings of ones self therapeutically. I can now look down on my history safely in the confident foundation that I have a love in my life, Rachel, who gives me strength, and I have a trust in God that is as sure and steadfast as an anchor in a storm.

I needed, in my adult life, to be able to find my childhood again and then work through my issues. It would be a therapy to eradicate the memories that flashed into my mind in idle moments. Perhaps I required an inner strength, needed to re-live the traumas and suicidal thoughts I felt when being the constant victim of my disability and a mentally unstable mother.

Life in a one-parent family, being dragged up in post war working class Salford is the thing sociologists and revolutionist's dream of. It was never my dream, just my nightmare, lived day in, day out as a child and hidden deep inside me until now. Now rapidly approaching my sixtieth year I can safely tell my story to you as my rehabilitation and righting of the many wrongs I felt I suffered.

It has not been written for you to enjoy or even to shock you. It has been written so that when we meet you may understand me a little better and why my personality is as it is today.

Reading or certainly reading for pleasure is not on my agenda, never has been, and never will be. Reading is not a pleasurable act even today. The letters of each word move around on the page so much that it gives me headaches. Very soon after beginning to read my brain gets irritable and restless hence getting down a full page is not easy. Letters when I write them with a pen fall into the words in different places and some get written back to front! Ask me why? No idea! But it sure as hell irritates me.

People have tried to read my writings since the tender

age of about 3 and it has caused me such self-doubt and a feeling of inadequacy all my life, even at times today! Some laugh when I send out information in Comic Sans, designers refuse to print in it. I find it to be one of the few type styles I can read. The letters do not move as much in it.

I have never read a novel from cover to cover in my life so it is not written copying any other style of influence. As for writing it, this book has taken nearly five years to complete, lots of hard work, headaches and hitting the F7 (spellcheck) button on the computer! I have significant Dyslexia and I need to get a grip of it. I needed to see what I can do and get on with that, rather than wallow in the pit of what I cannot and never will be able to do. Life before I discovered computers was one of almost illiteracy.

Illiteracy is so excluding in today's society. After much deliberation this book has been written and published specifically without a ghost writer or professional editor to correct my many mistakes.

Within the Book world I have had many authors, professionals and writers suggest that I put it into proper English. They suggested that instead of selling hundreds as it is, working the grammar correctly will enable it to sell thousands. Multi-national publishers will become interested in publishing it!

The Disability world people who have read it have a more pragmatic view. Statements such as 'Be true to yourself.' 'Let the world know how your disability affects you.' and 'It's all about your disability and keeping the writing as

Foreword

it is takes nothing away, only helps people see it through your disability.' helped me make the correct decision.

So, sorry if my English irritates you as you read it. I have at least 3 or 4 spelling mistakes each sentence. It is how my brain converts all it sees on paper and miss-converts the words I read in my silent reading. Being ejected from most English classes from Primary through to Secondary school also did not help. Need I say more?

This story is written just to explain, from my point of view, how my disability affected me in those dark days of closeted education and learning in days well before 'whistle blowing' on family cruelty by neighbours and friends who happen to witness a family in crisis. It's my therapy, but I do need to share it with others, it helps water it down and release the pain from within. Who knows, it may help others, please God.

My life today is much fulfilled and I am loved every day by Rachel. I hold a professional teaching post in a college for young people with disabilities which is extremely fulfilling and very time consuming!. The journey to get thus far has been very, very difficult.

Getting professional qualifications in Youth work, Nursing, Learning Support and then Teaching has caused me such stress. At times reading and writing is like wading up a fast flowing muddy stream up to my waist with a full and heavy rucksack on! I almost completed a Post Graduate qualification in Learning Disability at Manchester University which took me on the road to almost having another stroke. Such is the pressure put on me when I read and write. I now understand that having the trappings of academia is a false god to follow. The knowledge and some of the wisdom that comes with it is not. I have had three opportunities to attend my Graduations. I have not attended any. Inverted snobbery? Read on.

I thank you for allowing me to share it all with you. If it helps you to come to terms with issues in your life then all the agony of going back and reliving it all is worth every tear I have shed and each ounce of pain suffered.

Chris Stewart
Lancaster 2013

1

Beginning the Realisation

:The Tate Modern Art Therapy Course

The Child Psychologist is saying those words again. Why did I have to come on this course and suffer a professional kick back into my past? I buried my childhood along with my mother and father. I had immersed my past into the furthest part of my brain, the evil memories had been submerged in deep pools of ancient recall.

This is supposed to be an Art Therapy Course I'm on to help me support those youngsters with disabilities I work for. Instead it's more like a torture for me, the knife edges of pain which had spent years in concrete vaults within my head are now resurfacing.

These professionals, do they know that they are telling me that I'll have to go back to my inner child, the one that took all the pain and suffering, unravelling the torture I suffered. Look at my hands sweating, and legs all prickly, my heart is beating into the walls of my chest. They are only words he's saying, just words, but the power of the past is hitting my body in a way I feared it might. He is just explaining to the group but does he realise he's hitting me with such power because of my past? I never wanted it to happen, it scares me and yet excites me. How I wish I could be someone else, anyone else just someone normal. Even now at nearly sixty it just keeps coming back and haunting me.

Just like my disability, my past is not a blessing but a curse. Deep inside me in the labyrinth that is my history, I have demons, devils and pain, so much pain. It is masked by the facade I have as my outgoing personality but inwardly there is still pain, tears and hurt. Why do I have to rediscover it all again, to look at it, listen to it all and relive the life I have buried? My only redemption is that I bear no guilt or malice towards those perpetrators who wronged me so deeply. I have to do it.

"Just listen," he says to the group using professional therapy words like 'evil, reconciliation and deeply disturbed children' but does he really know it's me he's talking about. Does he know it? Is he looking at me? Can he see that he is twisting my innards into a tight knot? What do I do right now? Listen, go out, stare at the floor and give no eye contact or make a feeble excuse for the toilet.

Think Chris! Don't let your emotions get the better of you. Think in your head, hold your new wife Rachel in your arms as when you are alone in bed together and she is breathing next to you. Smell her, feel her chest moving slowly and her breath on your skin. The warmth she gives you will make it all go away, that deep feeling of being unconditionally loved.

Rachel gets me out of my past and holds me in love for today and in my future. I can see her now, feel her warm, soft, beautiful smooth skin and her smell. I'm holding on to her here in this training session although she is 60 miles away back in Lancaster. She makes me a real person, painless and good, deep inside. She is my shield against this verbal ploughing of my past.

My past, I can visualise mother's face etched into my deep consciousness; feel the torment of my tiny body helpless in her wrath. Never knowing when or how she would explode at my slightest misdoing. I can still feel the belt and the cold as I stand naked in the hall being nagged, my skin stopping the buckle when her temper erupts again. Another cut, legs aching, eyes red and tired, I just want sleep. Why does she do this? Why me? Can't I be someone else, live another life?

"Are you the evil one?" she screams at me. Do I really have the devil in me as she tells me so often?

Whatever I had done or not done, it was always my fault. Yes. Mother's right. She's now telling me how I should feel guilty for being not just bad and naughty, but evil and thick. I never learn, never ever listen, never sit still and never do as I am told. I can't write properly, read properly and I am just down right bad. I

3

have the devil in me!

It's true I can never spell and my writing is abysmal. I was just so naughty that I am evil. All my wrong doings were my entire fault as a child. This was drummed, hit and belted into me. Each hit going deeper than the skin that cut and bruised. The violence ingrained it into me until I would die believing it. Why can't I just be someone else? Just for a day. Here I sit today, having to go back and remember these terrible things but it is so hard.

Do this Chris, hold on to the vision of Rachel, she will save you, Don't let her go. God is also here saving me from my self-doubt, he has been here constantly throughout my life. But I must go back to the time of all my devils to exorcise them, then I can live and love freely without fear and pain.

I can kill them by writing about them and telling the world. Change it all from a secret to a transparent life. Tell all so others can understand who I am and why I am the person I am. Tell them about the curse I have and how it underpins all my behaviours. It's not an excuse for it but the reason, the real truth, no matter what mother said. I have to tell them I am not possessed as she constantly told me, I do not have the devil in me. I am a real, true, kind and emotional person who really wants to right wrongs and look out for those who are in need or need help.

My heart races again, he is saying the words that I know so well. He's describing me. What am I to do?

Can I really lay the devils of this curse to rest? Can I really tell my story? Do I tell about all the evil I was a victim of and the people who helped me through that were perhaps from the other side? No one will believe me, it's too complex.

I can't even write properly but all I have to do is remember what I did and what happened to me. Just write the facts and tell the world. I have to. It must be told.

Why spend so much time telling you about those sessions on that course? It was my initial and many formative years that were being stirred up. That period of my life was like an entire lifetime to me. A time that for so many years took away any innocence of childhood and formed the person I am.

I spent what seemed like an age regurgitating my own past on that course. Can I put my demons to rest with my writing? If so, they cannot be laid to rest in just a few sentences. This is the catalyst for what you are about to read. Through the Tate Modern Art Therapy Course I have the steel to sit and burn through my disability to write about my traumas in this book for you.

2

A Traumatic Birth

I do need to start at my birth. It's crucial for you to understand how I became disabled or blessed with my brain damage or personality. It was a very dark November night in 1952. How do I know? The tales from my two old aunts, Olga and Patty, still ring in my ears. Long dead now they revelled in telling me how I entered this earth, all the difficulties in keeping me alive and of course their part in the pantomime. Yes Pantomime for it was pantomime season in those dark days before Christmas and I was to play two central roles, the jester and those who are deemed as evil personified.

Let me take you to the tiny terraced house which had two coal fires lit, one down stairs and one in the front bedroom. This must have been a special occasion because there was only ever enough money to keep the downstairs one alight. Just two fires in the 100,000 that made this dirty old town of Salford so grim. The toxic fumes filled the air night and day in winter and the lungs of those poor souls who lived there in the gloomy northern town.

Little Alan was asleep in his bedroom at the rear of the house totally unaware that in the next room a life giving or maybe life threatening drama was unfolding. Little, because he was born so small and fragile, born too early and never quite caught up, size wise. He was placed on his father's arm just after he was born and his head fitted in the palm of Jim's hand. He was almost the weight of a bag of sugar. Alan struggled for life and yet managed to hold on to slowly grow into the bespectacled little four years old he now was.

If ever there was a daddy's boy he was the one, apple and pear of his father's eye. Poor soul, wore National Health glasses since he was 18 months old. Remember those little round ones that John Lennon made fashionable many moons later? Those glasses and his slight stature were the only visual sign that he struggled to grow and live in his initial days.

Now it was time for baby number two to arrive in the troubled Stewart family. Mother was in the bed next door shouting for and about her husband Jim. "Never bloody here when I need him. He thinks more of the bloody hospital and the Army than me."

Of course this was not dad's fault, he was working as a staff nurse on shifts that in those days were unchangeable. A mere staffy, no clout to ask Sister if he can change his working pattern. Long, long before the times where paternity leave is granted. You just had to let the women get on with it and hope you could hold a holiday and use it to cover seeing the wife and new child entering the world.

"Now come on, just think about getting baby out, breathe and push," Patty talked to mother with her soft northern accent. Patty and mother were two contrasting human beings, only related through mother's marriage to Jim and the thin line that joined them was ready to snap at any moment.

Patty was always called Patty and Jim knew her as the kind Aunt who lived next door but one, in Myrtle Grove, Weaste where he grew up. Mother despised her for her own reasons, which she never divulged to me in her life time. She also had issues with Olga, Patty's sister, again she never explained what these were to me or others in the family. Perhaps they both saw through her and might even have had the gall to tell my mother about her issues, who knows?

Mother lay on the bed writhing in agony swearing at the world and venting her annoyance at the man she had to marry. She was a small, thin almost a frail looking woman with dark red hair and pale skin. Her Aberdeen heritage was key to her looks, maybe her nurture was key to her insanities, who knows?

Her stature bellied her tenacity and she had the strength of three horses when angry. Mother called under her breath, between a moment of pain and pushing. Anger and pain. It just went together so naturally, and was the way life was to be for the little child about to be born.

Olga pulled Patsy, her sister, to one side. "Something's not right, I know it," she quietly whispered into her younger sibling's ear. The atmosphere in the small dimly lit room was getting as dark as it was outside. "This child should have been here long ago, we must try to get a doctor."

. Now calling out a doctor in those days was not a matter taken easily. Doctors were given a higher esteem in working society that sometimes they deserved, almost a reverence. But the situation was becoming grave.

Mother laid there, the sheets ringing in sweat from her traumas. She was not aware of the huddled discussions her in-laws were having. She just wanted rest and to get rid of the thing inside giving her the pain. The struggle of entering the world has never been easy. This time the child was stuck inside and not wanting to join humanity it was a prelude of his life to come.

The gas kettle screamed, it was dirty and tired from the heat that had made a thousand brews but ready with hot water for the new life. The steam rose from the bowl as Patsy climbed the steep narrow stairs, heating the skin on her face to double her feeling of anxiety. She was already hot inside and her face reflected her fears.

Mother was now giving some screams between her panting. "Come on child, come on!" Olga was sat side on the bed hovering over Mother's genital area trying to mop up the water from sheet with the towels before it soaked into the mattress.

The atmosphere was now intense enough to eliminate

all conversation between the sisters. They subconsciously knew the chance of losing both their sister in law and the unborn child was real. The silent glances between them was sufficient enough communication to share the gravity of the situation.

Olga stilled, "I think it's here," she mumbled under her breath. It must be dead, stuck so long in the neck of the womb. No life, no telltale signs of normality or what pass for normality in the process of giving up the world that had been so intimately its Mother for nine long months. Just screams from mother and a fear within Olga of a still born child.

"Its head is there!" Patty was excited and her voice reflected it, "Come on, just push for buggery, as hard as you can, just push and let it out."

Olga was more controlled and just wanted a closure to the sad episode. Glancing around the badly lit room she noticed the fire was glowing into embers. She wanted not to be there. Let the Doctor or midwife do this job, not her. She did not want the devils work of telling Mother the child was dead or a spastic. She knew the signs of still birth and was there just by circumstance. Life was cruel to her she contemplated. Not only did the Lord not allow her to have children of her own, she had to bring up some of her wayward eldest sister's children as her own and be a party to this terrible night of pain and sorrow.

The fire crackled as the raw coal fell on the glowing embers, smoke blew back into the room yet the three women were too preoccupied to worry about contaminating the air.

"The little sod is coming, it's nearly here," said Olga.

"Come on push harder," Patty replied.

"I bleeding well am, don't you start on me, you want to help then shut up and get a doctor."

Mother was in no position to dictate but she was angry enough to let it all out at her helpers. If only she had not listened to Jim and gone home that night of the nurses ball she would never have been trapped into this marriage through pregnancy.

Such shame and bitterness, how could she cope? Yet this second child will just an extension of the jail sentence she had to a man she never loved. A second child that is here only because she let him make love to her in a moment of fancy. Her fault and she was to pay the price.

The head began to appear; a rip signified that it was pushing out into the world, covered in blood. The bony mother stopped and panted, she cried softly as if in a daze, then screamed again.

"That bastard is never," she paused as if to get a strength from deep inside and breathed heavily twice, "coming anywhere near me again, I swear it!"

Olga was not listening, she held Mother's knees apart and watched the top of the child's head with grave concern. Thoughts ran through Olga's head. No movement and covered in blood, over twenty-four hours in labour now the end must be near, so near yet so far from being resolved.

"ARGGGGH," Mother yelled as the limp body slid out. The neck, then chest and legs all appeared in place but something was not right in the grand order of things. Olga could see the child was blue and had the cord wrapped around its neck. Lifeless it lay there on the bed but that instant seemed a lifetime.

Mother just lay panting and breathing as if having just run a marathon in an unfit body and with the weight of the world on her shoulder. For her she had. Patty lent over Mother and held her hand gently then whispered in her ear. "It's a boy, your Christopher and he has red hair just like Teddy did when he was born," Patty was a good honest soul but had just given Mother the words she did not want to know. Mother raised her head up a little and cursed.

"Another Stewart male into this world is another too bloody many," she dropped her tired head back onto the pillow and closed her eyes tight.

Why oh why could she not have the little girl she so desperately wanted. In her deep disappointment she had not noticed the lack of the first cry, that initial breath and shout that another life had entered this traumatic world.

Olga was worried, what was she to do; she stared at the lifeless thing in front of her. This was uncovered territory for her, a new and scary area she had no training or experience of, "Just move, cry, make out you are alive somehow," she thought. Patty leaned back and whispered to her kin,

"Quickly, untie the cord from around his neck, let him breathe and pick him up, smack him." She was fearful that they had lost precious seconds to get life into the boy.

Was he really dead or did he just want the kick start needed by so many precious bundles on entry from the secluded womb?

Olga just froze and watched as Patty gently but quickly lifted the 7 lb limp weight and wound the cord away from his neck. She then raised him up towards her shoulder and with the red, bloody head resting against her tired dress she smacked his tiny bottom cheeks with an almighty whack.

He still laid there a lifeless lump, only human in body but not in soul. She was to try again fearful that all her hopes of life would fade as she tried again to get him to enter the world of the living. Smack, the instant her motherly hand hit him again he jerked into life, coughed mucus out of his tiny mouth and cried.

It was a cry that seemed to ring across the dark, wet night, through the smoke and out into the world. Mother jolted back to reality.

"What colour hair has he got?" she questioned from out of her tears and with a fear hoping the fact given was wrong.

"Ginger of course," the proud aunt smiled as she wiped the little one down with a towel, "and he's just like his dad." True he had Ted's sandy hair. All his family called Jim, Christopher's father, Ted or Teddy, from the day he was born. Well when he came out all covered in a light ginger down what else would do but 'Teddy Bear'.

The newest Stewart was blue from the trauma that he suffered as he transcended the safe world of the womb to the battle ground he was to find in the real world but his hair was bright ginger. Patty jerked back into reality from the second respite following the last shout. The little boy seemed to stop breathing and living again. He was getting cold and his brief life seemed to be gradually slipping away again.

Patty could see the child was going blue again and needed warmth. Rapidly and silently she wrapped the tiny thing into a towel and moved him towards the fire. She was now in a race against the elements of winter to keep the precious body warm and alive. He was blue from lack of oxygen and needed to concentrate his tiny heart on keeping going, not fighting against any drop in temperature.

This little mite was not for living she thought. Yet she leaned over it, took the soulless body and lifted the poor wretch up her chest again. Quietly she peeled the towel away and "Whack!" she gave the smallest pair of buttocks in the room another hell of a smack!

This time the little hands moved again and the tiny head lent over to one side. "Waaaah." The tiniest wail filled the air of the dark room as his mouth opened and a tiny fist moved around his face into the gaping hole to suckle. Patty could now hold him and cuddle the babe without fear for his life. Gently she covered him again and held him over the fire for the additional warmth he required for his maintenance.

"Patty," Olga snapped "Get your coat on and go fetch the doctor. We can't keep this child alive without him." Mother snapped out of her daze, she just kept looking at the sleeping child laying in her arms.

"Get some brandy as well that should keep him warm inside, it's too bloody cold in here."

There was a growing panic as reality set in. This new child had been trapped by his life cord in the passage out of the womb and stopped breathing as he was trying to enter the world. He was known as a Blue Baby in common terms. It was as if he knew about the life he was to live and had rejected it before it began.

The two sisters had overseen his birth but were not the world's experts in midwifery, just two people who had the task thrust upon them by loose family bonds. Knowledge and experience were not the prerequisite for this roll, just blood ties. Obsessed as they were with keeping the child warm they did not relate to their sister in law until she moaned again on the birth bed.

"What is he like? Is he all right?" Mother quizzed after coming back out of her dazed condition.

"He just needs keeping warm," came the curt reply.

Patty then went downstairs into the dimly lit parlour. She knew where the posh sideboard was, back against the hall wall. The old Oak cupboard was always the starting place for any alcohol hunt and it was all too easy to release its prize.

"Brandy, that'll do," she muttered softly under her breath as she turned tail and scampered up to the front upstairs room again. The tiny short's glass quickly smelt of the life supporting alcohol and Olga took the glass.

"It'll do," she held it in one hand as she placed her little finger into the dark liquid. The smell drifted into the room and in a way it changed the atmosphere from the previous hours of tension and pain.

The child's purse mouth held the nectar for a few fleeting seconds on its mandarin slice like lips. They opened and he took into his body the first taste of this world he was to love and hate for the rest of his life. No choke, cough or splutter, just a faint whimper as if in submission to the life help he was getting. Maybe he was too tired after the exertions of his entry.

Olga tried again; the child reacted in the same way, so submissive and weak suckling on her finger. "My God," said Patty. "He sups like a good un, but the little bugger needs it." Turning her face to her younger sister, the spinster Olga looked deep into the eyes of the child holder.

"Will he be all right? I mean is there anything wrong with him? What do you think?" she whispered with a coldness in the meaning that chilled the room and took away any feeling near to joy and relief that had just passed.

"Yes, he's ok. Just get the sod to come as fast as he can." With that the older sister disappeared out of the room and moved down the stairs as fast as she could towards the door to summon the GP.

The child coughed and then started to cry after a lull that seemed bliss for the Aunt holding the weak bundle. She looked down and thought to the child.

"You are meant for this world and I'll make sure you stay here." With her free hand she poked into the fire. It roared into life the burning coal sending up its poison fumes up into the night air above and its life giving heat into the room. The extra heat made the new child's Aunt move back but keeping near enough to have the life saving warmth maintained on the babe.

Mother was still laid in her bed going between sleep and semi consciousness. She could hear Olga and Patty in their low mumblings but not understand what the centre of their conversation was about. She stirred in what seemed an age since producing her child to the world and giving up her final push with the scream to end all screams.

"Patty, can I have a look at him?" she tried to lift her head up but was exhausted from all her exertions and just fell backwards. Patty lent over her and placed the child beside her, he was whimpering and moving his mouth as if suckling at the breast.

"He smells like brandy," Mother retorted rather indignantly.

"Well I need to keep him warm till the doctor comes, warm inside. If you can think of anything better?" Patty gave back sharply. She stopped and thought about what she had said, instantly remorse flowed over her. She had not thought how Mother was or her needs, just the child once it had completed its journey into the world.

Troubled in his start and troubled in his life, there was no knowing on that night what lay in store for the child, his pain and heartache in the traumatic years ahead. He had survived and got over his first hurdle but had it left him with a lifelong legacy of disability? This first hurdle was just one with many more in front of him to scale.

3

The Horse and
Harrison's Dairy

Coke Street, Higher Broughton was on the edge of Salford. The next town adjoining it, Prestwich, was a world away. Its leafy streets and avenues were frequented by the Jewish community who worked their shops in Cheetham Hill, Manchester and spent the profits on large neat houses dotted across Prestwich.

Saturday was their holy day and most of the shops in Prestwich village were shut. A very strange experience for me, especially as I was brought up to regard Saturday as the main shopping day and Sunday as the day of rest, in fact almost complete shutdown. For the Jewish community Sunday was open house for working and selling and as I grew older I would sometimes frequent a bustling Cheetham Hill on a Sunday when the rest of Manchester was slumbering or shut.

Why I mention this odd little fact is because on many occasions mother would recall how, when I was a small baby and we lived in Higher Broughton, she worked every Saturday for three Jewish families just up the road in Prestwich, making and lighting their fires and setting table for them. She said all the family would walk to the Synagogue, leave the car on the drive, never work at all throughout the day only dress and eat. Saturday was defiantly their day of rest and mother's grafting meant she profited from it.

Do you have an initial, earliest memory? Go on stretch back and think of the very first thing you can uncover in the oldest corner of your mind. My first memory still stays with me today, clear as a bell ringing out over still water. I could not have been more than two, just a toddler. I was upstairs, looking out over the window sill of the back bedroom in the tiny terraced house in Coke Street.

My first memory was a horse, yes a horse, largest beast I had ever seen and it was there in our backing. A 'backing' is a local expression for the long walkway space between the backs of two sets of terraced houses. There in the middle of Salford, all terraces and mucky streets, a beautiful beast of the wild open plains. There, just passing my own back gate mysteriously left open as if set up for me to see this beast.

The sight must have been so shocking and so impressionable that it stayed stamped in my memory for all these years. A large chestnut brown beast that was bigger than any living thing I had ever seen or was to see for many years to come.

Many memories were to be etched into my miswired brain as if by acid into copper as I accumulated incidents and events in my early existence. This first one is as clear as the others and the animal theme was to run throughout my young life at least in my head if not in reality.

"Was this wonderful creature just a fantasy?" I must have thought. Was it to be just like the fantasy of the bird in the cage and the tin of paint I was to hold dear as my mechanism for survival in a cruel life? No, this beast was a reality. It slowly clomped up the cobbles as it walked towards the milk cart, feet covered in hair and large enough to carry it across any sand or snow.

You see at the end of the row of the tiny two up and two down houses that comprised Coke Street was the Harrison's Dairy. A little shop which sold all manner of dairy products, cheese, eggs and bread. It was a little shop but with a large stable behind and yard with a horse driven milk float in it.

There was a bell over the door that rang every time someone went in to the dingy little front room where people ordered items over a worn oak counter. The shop had a smell in it that came from another world. This aroma was produced from a concoction of milk products and the game, tied together at their tails, that hung over the counter.

Breath it in, go on, there was no other smell like it in the whole of Salford and it was there right at the end of my street. It was another world, a world that I could enter and escape in as a toddler. This must have been the start of my inner fantasies that became an inner reality for me. My escape mechanism from the bleakness and pain I was to endure. My fantasy world of birds in cages, animals in boxes and tins of paint was just beginning.

In those days, just after the war, to have a Dairy meant you had to have a horse to deliver the milk and farm produce with and that was what lived in the stable at the end of Coke Street, a real live horse. A horse to a child of two or three was such a mystical beast, especially right in the middle of this, dirty, industrial town.

Maybe it was the size of the animal or the smell it gave when the stable was being cleaned out that gave it a firm foundation in my memory bank. It was an awesome beast, moving so slowly along the cobbles the very ground resounding to the thud as it placed its foot down onto the entry floor. It whinnied as it moved past our back gate, adding to its rich mystery. A sound I had heard many times before from the stables but never seen its originator. Here before me was the creator, the very beast below, in my sight. That sound is one that carries me back into that moment whenever I hear it again.

In addition to this beast there was also was the mystical experience of visiting the shop and seeing the dead birds and the range of food, so rich when some things were still on ration and scarce.

The Harrison's themselves also added to the magic of the old shop. Mr Harrison was a thin man, always had a pipe from his mouth, never lit, just hanging there, used only for the occasional suck of the stale tobacco still left in it.

Only on very rare occasions now do I see a man smoking a pipe but I always ensure I walk around into the smoke to catch a breath of the past. It is a comforting smell, not related to the cancer bearing chemical mixture it really is, just a warm journey back into a comfortable part of my past.

His wife of some 40 odd years was generously proportioned and the opposite of the thin wire of a man. She always wore flowered dresses to her ankles and filled their moderate plump size. Never troubled, she would always have time to bend down and talk to the children who entered her magical world of commerce. She also had a soft northern voice, not brash but slightly polished in a non condescending way.

He never spoke, just sucked on the pipe and grunted an answer to any pleasantries offered him in conversation. The wink he gave from his deep brown eyes was communication enough to pass the warmth from his personality to you.

For a young whippersnapper like me the shop at the end of our street was such a marvellous place with scary and fascinating things to see and smell. A truly multi sensory experience, long before the advent of high tech rooms to produce a similar arousal of the senses.

Harrison's Dairy, it was a grotto of experience that will be forever etched into my mind. After all the bleakness of war and near starvation rations to have such a kaleidoscope of such fantasies right here on my doorstop was richness indeed.

4

Stonegate Drive

We must have moved to Stonegate Drive, Swinton soon after my magical encounter with the horse because I cannot remember any more of the dingy terraced house in Coke Street.

Stonegate Drive was all that Coke Street was not. It was a newly built semi-detached house in a spacious suburb of Manchester, called Swinton. In those days Swinton was next to Salford but not a part of it. The house was in a quiet cul-de-sac, so far away from the grime of Higher Broughton and Weaste, it should have been idyllic.

We even had two small neat little gardens, one at the front and one at the rear. These little green areas were to be the first piece in the jigsaw I built up when escaping from the traumas of life, escape into the world of nature and an environment that I could soak into without fear of pain and anger.

The house was also a supposed to be an aspiration for any married couple especially for their two young boys to grow up in. There was a small enamelled range fire in the back room which heated up the water and an electric cooker, with no gas in the house, it was so modern. No double glazing, not invented then, just metal window frames due to the lack of wood available at that time.

Mother always called Stonegate drive 'Jerry built', not quite sure what she meant at the time but I later understood completely it's meaning for shoddy workmanship. Yet this was held out to be the ideal home in the New Britain.

Seen now on the old news clips it smacked of the emergence of prosperity after the restrictions of the war years. A new world, a new start, yet behind the net curtains the horrors which were inflicted in the life of this child was to be ignored by neighbours and family. Why, oh why when the façade was so positive did the house and family life only mirror themselves in a grotesque parody?

Dad, now a fully qualified male nurse, had landed himself a job at Hope Hospital on the other side of the dirty old town. The Swinton house was a lot nearer his roots than Higher Broughton and yet allowed him the luxury of being able to choose a nearly new semi to buy in a much sort after part of Manchester.

Yet underneath this gossamer thin lie of normality and success was, in our house, a world of hatred, broken relationships and cruelty. Cruelty that was first between my parents to each other then transferred by mother and vented onto her children. I was the middle child, bearing the brunt of her venom for all of my formative years. My older brother left Stonegate Drive as soon as he could after his traumatic time when dad left.

Having a girl was always mother's dream. Margaret, my beloved sister, appeared four years after me and she was unwittingly placed on a pedestal by mother. Such a position came back to haunt her later in her adulthood but as a child she led a different life to me within the same four walls.

This house was to be a cold, naked place for me where I yearned to leave either by ordinary methods or by removing myself from this life to a higher, better one. My support in times of turmoil were often the supernatural little people who talked to me from the other side until my sister was old enough to give me her devotion and love as a sibling. God also stayed alongside me. My discussions and confessions to him, through my tears, meant that I knew he was always watching, waiting for me to jump into the safety of his arms.

5

The Knife Attack

My troubled mind can always summon up the horror of that night, probably my first memory of Stonegate Drive. Whether my younger sister Margaret was born or not I cannot remember but the picture is as sharp as the kitchen knife used.

Alan and I must have been awakened from our sleep by the noise of the fight. Alan shook me into semi awareness. "Hey, wake up, they are fighting again. What shall we do?"

Instantly I felt the 'flight or fight' rush. I cannot have been more than four but there was an adrenaline pump in my little system that rarely comes over someone unless in extreme moments. It is a psychological rush that can be converted into a physical power to lift cars up or move mountains. This night I just felt it but did not use it.

Alan and I both scrambled out of the old three-quarter

bed we struggled to share and rushed into the larger bedroom next to ours at the front of the house where the sounds of the argument was coming from. I say argument, this was not one of the normal ill feeling conversations between both my parents that passed as their norm for communication. Mother was screaming and Dad shouting and both parents were swearing very loudly. No other noise, no pots thrown hitting the wall, no doors slamming, no glass breaking, there was just abusive language at full volume.

We ran pushing the door open and then both stopped dead in our tracks. In the semi darkness from the street light that came through the cheap curtains we could see a scene of fear that hit Alan and I into numbness. The image of your own father kneeling over your mother on the bed, holding a knife at her throat and with a wild look on his face sends a cold shiver into you and stops your normal reactions from working. It still haunts me today as I can so vividly recall the incident.

As much as I hated my mother, this ran far into my subconscious as fear and a deep feeling of hopelessness. I knew I was witnessing a trauma, a wrong and something fearful. A simple question ran through my tiny mind. Was he going to kill her?

"You drove me to this, you bitch," he yelled in the semi darkness. Then she laughed back into his face in a manic sort of a way.

"Go on, kill me in front of the children, and let them see what kind of a man you are then eh!" Alan and I both cried, no, yelled out in panic.

"Don't do it dad. DON'T DO IT!" he looked across at us both and then slapped mother hard.

"You drive me mad, why do you do it, you're a bloody nutter."

With a heavy clout he sent the back of his hand across her face. Her head turned away from us with the strength of the blow then she turned back to look her husband in the eye. She laughed, yes laughed in his face then spat at him a spit so accurate from only inches away. He yelled.

"You bastard!" he leapt off her wiping her spittle of his face with the eiderdown. We still stood not moving.

"That's the type of man your father is," she hurled at us. I stood there in silence, no words would come out right, and then I just cried. Neither Alan nor I could do anything. It did not have to be like this but it was and we just stood there helpless watching the traumatic events just a few feet away.

We both just cried and cried running back into our room slamming the door behind us as if we could to keep the evil outside. No remorse, no explanation, both Alan and I were just left with the festering memory and fear of the 'What next?'

Listening in the night stillness for another chapter to unfold we lay on our bed, not holding each other for comfort, just separately, back to back, within our deepest thoughts and traumas. I went to sleep crying into my pillow.

This was to become a familiar way for me to slide from the uncomfortable reality of the life I received into the often short respite known as sleep. Dad slept on the couch downstairs that night and was gone, off to work in the morning by the time I got up. Mother did not mention it again right away just referred to the incident on occasions as the example of 'What kind of a father you have!'

• • •

"My words won't come out right, I feel like I'm drowning
I'm feeling weak now, but I can't show my weakness
I sometimes wonder where do we go from here.
It doesn't have to be like this."

Beth Moulam. Aged 12

6

My Brother Alan and I

My brother Alan and I always had an uneasy relationship from when I was aged four onwards till he left abruptly at fifteen. He so badly missed his dad after he had been thrown out by mother. This draw eventually resulted in Alan running away from home as a very young teenager, leaving to find his father.

Aged around fifteen he left Stonegate Drive and lived in digs. He saw his father on a regular basis and did not contact his mother. The lack of any bond between us which ensued I must admit I did not help with, but tough as I thought I was, I had times of weakness that Alan exploited.

Sometimes he gave me an additional layer of guilt, hurt, pain and blame that was piled on top of those already regularly serviced by my mother. I hated him for it, I could vent my anger on him in fist fights which I could never do with the all powerful villain of the home, the real target of my retaliation, Mother.

On reflection Alan did have a purpose in my life, he was my literal punch bag that I could work up a sweat of anger with and release pent up feelings into his body at the end of my fists. Now it's all different, he's just my brother again, distant as the miles across the Atlantic make it, he's just a shy retiring guy who releases his love for others by working with youngsters, coaching into them soccer skills in his spare time.

I can say now I love him even with this distance making us not see each other. When we do meet and hug, it is in the historic knowledge of caressing away the pain we inflicted on each other. This warmth is such a far cry from those incidents of hatred and loathing we both went through as confused and hurt young children.

Bed wetting is nowadays seen as a normal but embarrassing phase a child can go through. If extended over a time period, other signs of distress are looked for. How the world has changed.

Alan and I slept in a three quarter size bed on a second hand mattress which was not sprung but filed with cotton or similarly uncomfortable material. No memory foam comfort filled, full and complete nights sleep was to be had on this one. No place for a spillage of urine to drain off or dry on this old style back ache inducing lumpy mattress!

I vividly recall the night I wet the bed, an infrequent occurrence I like to think, but this particular night I really did open my bladder nocturnally, and opened it very wide! Alan woke me with such a hard poke, a kick in my back intended to make me gain instant consciousness. I startled and right away knew what was wrong. The stench and warm, wet sheets gave my brain no time to contemplate any other scenario.

He virtually pushed me out of bed, kicking me with his foot in my back, quietly uttering derogative curses about how I was a baby, and how mother would kill us both if she found out. We worked hard for the next hour or so in the dark and cold of the room, rubbing the sheets with the luke warm hot water bottle in a desperate attempt to remove the evidence. The sheets had soon gone cold with the exposure to the night air in the unheated room and the wet surface I had produced. Eventually we gave up trying to rectify the problem and hid the sheets in the airing cupboard and slept under the old, feather filled eiderdown.

All this going on was with the light off, in case she heard its loud click and with my sibling continually cursing and swearing at me in quiet, low tones. What was I to do? I felt cold, tired and very ashamed, totally to blame knowing we were only a faint sound away from deep pain and trauma if she cottoned on to our misfortune.

Bed time was not necessarily a time of respite from the evil overlooking of mother. You see Alan and I were always sent up together at 7pm and later 8pm. This instantly created an animosity between us. I mean can you name two children with a four year age gap who still have the same bed times? Alan rightly so, was aggrieved for years about this and often released his anger at the injustice on me once we had gone up stairs. This relieving of annoyance was capped by the threat of Mother hearing us fight.

We also sometimes put the bedroom light on to read, another activity that could lead to the mental torture of being nagged for hours or hit with the belt. The house was still wired with the original big heavy light switches fitted during construction, just after the war. They stuck out from the wall at 90 degrees, could draw blood if you caught the side of our head on them and when switched on or off went with a mighty "Thump!"

This thump could be heard in the evening throughout the house when it was quiet and mother was downstairs. We tried to deaden the sound by covering it with the pillow but no, "THUD," it would send an alarm downstairs that we had been reading with the light on. It was the trigger for her to exert her authority! According to mother, going to bed was only for getting to sleep and woe betide anyone of us who defied that or any other of her rules.

For some reason she had a great aversion to us reading or talking when in that bedroom. I remember one time Alan had one of the new little transistor radios and he would often listen to radio Luxemburg under the sheets, until the night he was caught! A good thrashing and confiscation was the key for children not doing as they were told, according to her.

7

Tin of Paint in the Cartoon House

Before dad left for good we spent an occasional Saturday of drab ordinariness as a family in Manchester shopping. All four or five of us (when Margaret had arrived) would go. We were dragged around immense department stores which were no fun for me but the promise of a visit to the cartoon cinema treat was worth waiting for.

Saying they were no fun I do recall being fully engaged when we were in Lewis's, the largest department store in town. They had lifts that took you up and down the various floors of the gigantic building. Not the slick self service, talk to you and mirrored units we have today but old cranky ones with steel folding doors that always had a man to operate them.

Not just any man but a special type of human. They always seemed to be war heroes. They would have a smart uniform on and perhaps an arm or leg missing. Yes it seemed that the war hero's that came home missing a limb could always get work in those days as lift operators in large department stores. Their missing limb would be noticeable by the neatly ironed uniform and it's carefully tucked in empty sleeve or trouser leg, so conscious and a damming statement of their heroics for King and country.

I know that I always looked, probably so ignorantly in a child like way, but with such awe, never talking to them just wondering what had befallen them to have such harm done to their bodies. They did speak as the vertical motion halted and they lent forward to open the steel mesh gates, explaining what was on the floor we had just arrived at.

"First floor, ladies clothes and underwear, men's dressings." Men's dressings? I used to think, what are they doing, getting up late or wearing dresses? Was it for other war heros with only one limb? Did I have to go through such pain and trauma of battle and losing a limb before I could get the job of being a 'lift man'? Such was a little child's thoughts and memories of the aftermath of war so visible to all. Disability in those day was well hidden in hospitals and without today's mobility so when it hit me in the face, I just absorbed it visually, never questioning or querying it.

I was always kept engaged by the thoughts of the men who operated the lift. How did the Nazi's blow them up? Were they going out of a foxhole, charging to glory then get a stray bullet? Were their best friends killed and they had to carry the body back to the medics, getting a bullet whilst being a hero? A thousand questions floating around my little head filling me with excitement and awe. This kept me focused until the end of the shopping, then an hour of another imaginary paradise was to come.

In town there was a particular cinema that only played cartoons, a continual show from early morning till late repeating the show every hour. It was my imagination that topped up my extra sensory ideas as a child, respite from the horrors of living as Christopher Stewart. Part of my life, part of my imagination, part of my escape, was that I had imaginary friends that I could carry around, talk to and intercourse with other sane humans about them.

Not only did I have one but a full repertoire, of, a Bird in a cage, a box with an endless stream of small animals in, dependent upon where I would be or who I would ask for it to be kept safe with. Then there was my favourite friend, a tin of paint.

Each played their part in my sanity. That particular day I had faithfully and diligently carried my imaginary friend, the tin of paint, all the way up Partington Lane to the bus stop outside the Town Hall, on the bus into Manchester and best of all around each and every department store. Wow did my arms ache! I even managed to store it under the table of the UCP cafe upstairs on Market Street whilst we had a drink as respite from mingling in the crowds.

Of course it was ludicrous for me to take a full tin of paint, imaginary or otherwise into a cinema to watch cartoons. It was so dark in the pictures I would probably forget it. So what did I have to do with it? Well the cinema, in my best memory, was from the outside a rounded building, covered with light brown tiles to give an air of opulence and style. There was one of those old curved entrances with glass doors, lots of brass accessories, inside were polished wood doors and marble floors. I gently placed my tin of paint carefully behind one of the open glass doors, hooked back on to the wall with a polished brass hook. The commissionaire was busy talking to another customer and I was quick enough to not let him see my friend being left by me quietly, just behind the door.

Soon I was absorbed into the carton show peacefully knowing that the family eruptions were not to take place for at least the next hour. Wow, a full hour of disengaging from the realities and horrors. Cartoons, with fun and laughter in them, full of such talking animals, all given life on the large screen. Newsreels that seemed to me slightly boring and an intermission from the colourful sketched hero's I loved. It was only to be ended with, "This is where we came in let's go and get the bus." Life at that age can be instantly changed or dictated by such a simple catch phrase.

Off we trouped, no light conversation between any of us, just the silence of 4 individuals walking together. Half way down the busy street my mind bolted me into the horror of the situation that I had just created. I had left my tin of paint behind! "My paint tin, I've left my tin of paint behind the door," I cried and vividly remember the instant argument of blame and counter blame that passed for communication between my mother and father.

"You go back for it," she retorted.

"No you go, I've got the bags!" he replied curtly. Quickly she streamed back.

"You don't want any of your hospital friends to know your child has imaginary tins of paint do you?"

"Bloody hell I'll go for it then," he stormed off back to the Victorian façade that was holding my best friend in waiting till father rescued it. As he lent in, in full view of my eagle eyes, to lift up the imaginary tin he attracted the attention of the huge figure in the purple uniform, the commissionaire.

"What are you doing?" he bellowed.

"Just getting this tin of paint," came the meek reply as dad lifted the thin air handle holding the non-existent paint tin. A strained silence ended with the stern look the commissionaire gave him.

Puffing and red faced father marched down the street, in full view of the many shoppers holding at half arms length my pride and joy. Was I the only person in the whole of Manchester to see my friend, full of gloss paint and not a bit spilt? He thrust his empty fist into my hand and finished his embarrassing moment with a, "You bring it to town again and I'll bloody have you."

I don't recall Dad living with us much longer after that but I don't think it was as a direct consequence of my vivid imagination and collection of bird cages and tins of paint!

8

Taking my Pets Around

I did have adult people in the real world that I thought saw my imaginary pets as my friends and even helped me to care for them. Many a bus conductor would have a lengthy conversation with me as I sat alongside the open doorway on the downstairs of the Corporation Transport bus. Bus conductors, in their idle moments, after collecting fares and waiting to shout the next stop to the passengers would stand in the open area where passengers hopped on and off the bus. No doors to protect people from the cold and wet, just a long silver bar to hold on to as the buses trundled around Greater Manchester.

Each conductor would stand facing the open space and ring the bell hidden under the stairs to the top deck that was behind them. For many years I would wonder how the bell would ring, not knowing it was being pressed by a hand behind their back under the stair well, in the space where the cases went.

The conductors would often ask what I had in my hand, held so carefully and at arm's reach. Once explained they would then pass comments with me about my tin of paint or parrot on the long journey to an aunt's across Manchester or into town for half a day's shopping. These guys spent all their working lives shouting out the stops and sometimes giving some humorous or directive comments about the next stop. Talking to a passenger so small would be just a piece of cake to them and help fill their working day with a little distraction.

There was also the shop staff who worked in the Coop just around the corner who often asked me how I was and what was I carrying today when I was in shopping for the basics with mother. Originally the Coop was a large open shop with lots of wooden cupboards and shelves behind the enormous counters which encompassed the edges of the area and held the large polished metal till. There was a hand operated slicer on the meat section, bright red paint and chrome that was kept spotlessly clean and made a swishing noise when being expertly and so carefully operated by staff.

Your food order was placed into your shopping basket as it was being positioned together from the list compiled on a note pad from mother's verbal instructions. The staff wore stainless white coats and had sharpened pencils behind their ears to count up your order with. It was a few years after moving to Swinton before the shop was 'converted' into a mini supermarket and was one of the first of its kind in Salford.

The shop staff were now sitting at smart modern tills next to the door which replaced the large counters and ancient till. Foodstuff was placed on open access shelves in isles around the floor space. Little wire baskets were picked up at the entrance on the left by its shoppers who had to select their goods themselves. The door on the right was reserved for the exit only.

There was now no room for the old chair where frail or tired customers used to sit on while waiting their turn or time for the chat about family matters the staff used to spend their time doing whilst serving you, listening and chatting. Speed was now of the essence and progress dictated that some social niceties were left behind in the quest for a quicker turnaround of shoppers, goods and money.

This mini supermarket was a totally new experience for mother and I when we went in, it was deemed 'the future'. Unfortunately the conversion lost that friendly feeling, perhaps thrown out with the old fittings and large polished metal till that went 'ding' as it was opened and money transferred into it. The dividend was still the same but the heart of the shop had taken a beating. The familiar faces who asked me about my imaginary pets had faded away when the refit came. Incidentally it lay empty the last time I drove past its doors on Partington Lane on one of my infrequent visits back to Swinton.

Now the lady, who kept the tiny Off Licence, on the

other side of Partington Lane, was my favourite shop person of all. I cannot remember her name but in those days I trusted her because she totally believed in me, or so I thought at the time. She would always ask what I had in my hand, be it a bird, animal or what colour tin of paint. She would never smirk or laugh when I explained what imaginary item I was holding aloft with in my hand.

The tiny shop she owned on Partington Lane was crammed with all manner of items and had a large long glass fronted fridge portioning the counter from the rest of the shop. She was open from early each day till ten at night. Its extra special feature was it opened on Sunday when all the rest of Swinton was closed, a real convenience store.

The whole shop was crammed into what was the front room of the cottage, set in the middle of the row of terraced houses. Rows of glass jars inside displayed their contents of multicoloured sweets high on the shelves. The one exception from the glass was the large metal tin of Uncle Joe's Mint Balls which travelled all the way from Wigan. The picture of 'Uncle Joe' is still used today on the front of the tins and is a relic left intact from my childhood. Meat was displayed in another large glass fronted fridge which also housed pies and other such luxuries. Mother would be a frequent visitor for half a pound of sliced ham and a white sliced loaf.

The daily deliveries of pies were initially piled next to the bread, stacked on the side, most of which came in a grease proof paper wrap. This wrapping was a bonus for me when the bread was finished as I could place it under my bottom and held at the front as I travelled down the local park slides to make my journey back to terra firma so much quicker. This was another skill of mine that would occasionally back fire when I had made the slide far too fast by overuse of the grease proof paper!

Hurtling headlong down with no way of breaking or slowing the speed I sometimes kept on sliding when the metal structure had ended. This led to another bruising of my frail body and either my backside or nose could encounter grit and stones with a force of friction it was not meant to do, ouch! Good fun though and was a thrill for me until my pants got ripped then I had to suffer the consequences back at home.

My favourite stock item to eat from this little shop were the Ducks, peas and potatoes sweets she kept in a large glass jar ready to be weighed on the white scales and poured into little paper bags from the silver dish. Saying that, I did have a great fondness for eating raw jelly as a child! It was the kind that came in blocks, its little squares ready to be ripped off and plonked into a bowl of boiling water. I loved it raw and would often steal some from the kitchen cupboard hoping the one piece taken would not be sufficient for her to notice, delicious.

The lady back in the shop would serve and chat to customers over the top of a wooden pull up counter next to the till and right in front of the door into the back room. Whenever I would call in with mother for her bread or a half pound of sliced ham the shop keeper would readily offer to keep which ever little friend I was carrying behind the counter for me. I agreed every time and she would carefully and gently lift my imaginary package up over the counter and then rest it behind her wooden lift up counter. I could walk home assured that my friend would be safe until I returned to collect it. Once collected again I could then carry it around and care for it as was my want until the next time it needed a refuge.

Today I wonder if any of the aggressive sales courses delivered by large multinational conglomerates have a section on 'Looking after imaginary pets overnight for customer's offbeat children' in them. It worked for me and I always tried to keep my custom in that shop over the years, following her little acts of kindness. Fortune has since smiled upon me and I quietly stopped this particular trait of carrying imaginary pets and paint as I grew up and progressed into the juniors!

● ● ●

"I believe in myself, I can do anything if I want!"

Beth Moulam aged 12

9

Early Holidays With Dad

Despite the fractional family ethos I can remember there were two holidays we all had together when dad was still at home. The first was in a caravan at Rhyll, Wincupps to be precise, around the time I was in primary school. Imagine after the existence we had, to be taken away and spend time on holiday by the sea was such a jolt from the blue. A cousin of ours, Mothers brother's son, from Weybridge, came and as he was in his mid teens it must have kept the parental fighting to a minimum. The journey was eventful enough and I recall a friend of dad, I think he was called Jack, drove us there.

I call him Jack, because that was the general name dad used at home for nearly all the males he had an acquaintance with. I remember a man called Jack turning up at our house to redress the pointing and sort out the brickwork at home and he said he was asked to by dad. Mother never let him in because she had not been told first by my dad. She went berserk when he landed home.

"Jack! Jack! They're all called bloody Jack! Why don't you tell me first when they are to land? I'm not letting anyone in that I don't know and I know they're all called Jack."

There were a lot of other words said in anger but those I cannot remember, probably because I went upstairs and hid in my bedroom, listening to the dulled words in the argument below. Yes calling other men "Jack" was one of Dads traits. It was just another aspect of his personality in her mind that annoyed her and drove Mother to nagging point.

In the late Fifties family cars were few and far between so to have a friend with a car must have been quite a plus point. To have one that was an estate, or 'Shooting Break', would have been even better. It was a Hillman Minx estate to be precise, a big bulbous thing that plodded along the country roads pre motorway and took us over the border to Wales and our holiday.

It had four doors and the back window was a door that opened to gain entrance onto the space for suitcases. We all packed into it, cases, Mother and Dad, our cousin, Alan, Margaret the baby and of course me with 'Jack' driving. I remember it so well because I was tucked into the back part of the estate with the cases and kept feeling sick.

So much for a quick, straight through journey, more like a stop start, in and out of the back to vomit, escapade. It was my very first holiday I remember and no matter what else happened on that week away I can only but always vividly recall two things about it.

Funny thing is how I, as a small child, related more to the sensory aspects of the caravan than any other feature of the holiday. No trip out or times spent on the beach, arcades, fairgrounds or running into and back out of the sea, chasing each wave of the tide. What elements are ingrained to rediscover some half a century later? The sand on my feet or between my small toes, smelling Candy Floss for the first time, lights of the arcade, salt water and sea air?

No! The most indelible elements were in the caravan, an old well worn five berth brown thing probably built in the just after the war period. It was the first time I can recall using Gas as a heating or cooking fuel and the bottled gas has a perfumery of its own. I can still smell the gas rings and fire used to cook and warm the van. It was the very first time I had seen or heard gas, Stonegate Drive was all electric as the ultra modern houses were and Coke Street's fittings did not hold in my memory box.

It was exciting for me to see the naked heat under the kettle and hear the noise it made. Gas from the bottle also gave the caravan a smell that I had never experienced before. It is a smell that goes into the memory bank of childhood smells. It sits alongside the peculiar smell that your old Aunts house has or when certain foods are served up only on special occasions even of say Old Spice on an aging man. You know the smell that you cannot describe but hits you when you unexpectedly come into contact with it again. Today we are fortunate to have a small caravan used for holidays in Picardy, France which still rekindles these memories when I light the small gas stove for the washing up water.

The other experience I hold on to, well, you would never guess in a month of Sunday's. Go on, try to imagine that caravan holiday and guess what it was that I still vividly recall. It was the strangest feeling, again held on to today and still relights my history. I thought I was living almost outside, the nearest I had ever come to sleeping under the stars. Heaven was only a thin sheet of aluminium away. It was marvellous.

Every evening I listened to the sound of the rain on the caravan roof. Yes, pattering Welsh rain on the aluminium sheet roof. The fact that it was supposed to be a holiday and have buckets full of sunshine did not enter the equation. I just wanted to listen to the buckets full of rain pattering above my head. Not dramatic in the vast scheme of things but just the same I revelled in it. Never before had I had such a close encounter with nature whilst in bed or on the toilet or having my breakfast.

This holiday held, for me, experiences that my dreams were made of and made my dreams for me. It was captured in my sensory inner so deep rooted that I can pull it out and recall it whenever I want to. Why can I recollect with such detail images like this yet tell me your name and moments later I've forgotten it? It is said my brain is miss-wired, misfiring more like, spasmodic in the way it learns, remembers and unscrambles the everyday coding we call communication. What I would not have given to be 'normal' yet almost treasure a small number of the memories I can recall.

The second and last holiday we had together as a family was at Pontin's Holiday Camp, Middleton Sands, Morecambe. How long it was after the first I do not know, the times seemed to be fuzzily fused together then with no real clear cut separations. They are just like film clips joined together, triggered by a smell or word or memory, not a play button that starts at the beginning runs its course in time zones and finishes at the right time. I was certainly at school, Margaret was a toddler so I would be about five, six or even seven.

Getting to the Morecambe holiday camp entailed a long train journey up the Lancashire coast to the edge of Morecambe bay. Arriving at the small but beautiful Edwardian Morecambe Railway Station I was in awe at the view as I clambered up the open topped Double Decker bus outside that was contracted to take us all to the beach side holiday camp a few miles out of town.

I left the station and could see right across the bay to the Lake District. Wow, it was a bay that followed the eye line and kissed the other side of the world where the mountains were. Beautiful tall almost purple mountains that I could dream of climbing, and having a thousand adventurers upon like herding sheep and living in tents or in small caves. This visual delight hit me like an art critic seeing an old master for the first time. Living in this area now I still never tire of the view across the bay.

Even mundane activities, such as shopping on the front at Morecambe, with the fabulous views, still has the deep respect of this dirty city born dweller. The consistent rain in this Bay area is not really an issue to me, especially as I hail from Manchester, no pun intended!

I must have been a lot older at Middleton Sands than the Rhyll holiday as so many aspects can be remembered in my long term box of recollections. I remember so much more detail around this week's break. Travelling upstairs on the bus, open topped, I could also see over fields and farms as we travelled along the narrow country roads to the oasis of entertainment and respite. There in the distance appeared what looked like a vast ocean liner moored alongside hundreds of chalets and holiday flats.

The bus rumbled nearer and I saw a sight I could never had imagined even in my wildest fantasies. It was a large complex build right in the middle of the camp in the form of a sea going cruise ship. This was mind boggling for me. It was to me a real ship, a cruise to America or India, such luxury, especially to one who lived off such a poor diet and used his imagination to create a world to remove him from his reality. Would I be spending a full week, albeit with him and her arguing, in such a wonder land?

I could not hold on to my excitement. I already did not want this holiday to end, and I had not departed from the bus yet! Was it to live up to its promise I had seen on initial contact? Here was a place where I could play in the parks and on the beach on my own in safety and without the fear of being chastised.

Each evening the blue coats would have a bevy of entertainment for us in what was the dining room by day and a night club by night. That week we never ventured off the camp, never needing to, for it was all there, on tap for us to soak up.

I do poignantly remember that we had two chalets, little wooden affairs but big enough to stable me in my tiredness to recharge my batteries for the next day's playtime. Dad, Alan and I slept in one and Mother with Margaret in the other. There was obviously something very not right with their relationship then but I was oblivious to all this for the week as I could fill my time with more important matters.

A new adventure I encountered was entering competitions. I pursued them with an eagerness to win and prove myself to be a star. First of all I went in to the Strong Man competition, and guess what? Came nowhere! My puny little frame with knots on cotton was no match for the older boys who kept fit, swam, played football and worked out. Parading around the swimming pool with arms lifted in a biceps bulging pose was wasted on my stick like limbs. The laughter I got as I paraded around for the judges was patronising but back then I thought it was all part of the competition.

I also entered the fancy dress as a packet of Capstan Cigarettes. I just found a large cardboard box that the cigarettes came in and cut a hole in each side for my arms. I was pleased as punch with it. There was even an unlit

51

cigarette hanging from my mouth borrowed from Dad. Wow, now I was going to win the voucher for the shop and guess where I came in the grand competition? Yes, another resounding absolutely nowhere! I was surprised and even felt sad for a short while.

Soon I eroded my sorrowful feelings of despondency when I clambered aboard the old static Fire engine next to the play ground. This ancient relic was used as an activity for the countless adventurous boys like me. In my head it took me away to many emergencies. I put out countless fires with imaginary hoses and water saving babies from burning windows and carrying old ladies down fiery inferno filled stairs.

In the evenings all our fractional family trooped in to the large restaurant cum ballroom to listen to the dance bands and watch the entertainment. Closing my eyes I thought I could be boarding a ship sailing the tropical seas, living life as a rich, posh person with a family who did not fight and argue and had lots of money.

I remember dad giving me a drink from his pint and mother calling him rotten for it. It was embarrassing for us all but mother kept on. We left early that night, dad walking back the chalet being barracked from behind by her for behaving in such a manner.

Irrespective of that incident life for me that week was almost utopia. How soon it was to end. The trip back to Morecambe station on the open topped bus was filled with a sadness in me that had not been there when I arrived in such a state of awe and wonder.

As Saturday came around we went back to our routine lives back in Swinton, living with the constant arguing and fighting between Mother and Dad. This cycle was to end thought when he was thrown out one day having given mother the news he was to be promoted and to work nights at Hope Hospital.

"Nights!" she bellowed at the news. "No father and husband works nights!" With that she went upstairs and threw his clothes on to the front lawn. We, the children cried, he left and Mother got worse not having the lid kept on her imbalances by having my Dad around.

Dad moving out heralded a new chapter in my life with a violent and mentally unstable mother. She was soon to start directing her hate and anger towards her children which I was to endure for the next ten years or so. Dad could physically stand up for himself but we small children were totally subject to her ranting and enforcement of discipline as she saw fit.

We spent a lifetime growing up, held in fear which forced Alan to take drastic measures to escape and made Margaret emigrate as soon as she was old enough to. For my part this dramatic lunge in our lives drove me further into the fantasy world I used for survival but it also gave me an insight to another world, one beyond earthly realms.

Was this God sent or just my imagination? Contact from beyond was not imagined by me at the time. It took a medium to make me realise that the spirit world would be a part of what help kept me conscious, sane and safe.

10

My Troubles in the Infants

Another journey I took as a child was so full of incident and trauma that it really deserves another book but I will try to condense it to just a chapter in my fight both against and for my self-preservation. This chapter runs alongside life at home but actually starts at my birth. It is the sudden realisation of what can only be termed as my handicapping which I was labelled with when I ran into 'education'.

My 'Not fitting any hole that society has for us to comfortably fit into,' began to become apparent when I started Primary school! Moorside County Infant and Junior School to giver it its full title. It is a very large school, about eight hundred pupils I think, with a few famed ex pupils. One who frequented it at the time when I was there was known as Dr Banshee's lad, later to become the actor Ben Kingsley. He was a lot older than me but his notoriety at the time was that he was the only coloured person in the whole of the school. This made his presence even more memorable. A certain footballer, Ryan Giggs, followed him later, well after my time. One ex pupil was to become famous the other both famous AND infamous in his later life, and then there was me; infamous only in my life during school!

The first I knew I was seen as different in the world outside my home was when, in very early infants, my left hand became the initial part of my physical being to be connected with my curse. Teachers sat us all in neat rows pupils coupled in the old joined wooden desks. Open plan had not been invented then and we followed the time honoured Victorian system of uniformity. The well worn wood housed an ink well and the lid of the desk hinged up so books and pencils could be housed out of the way.

I actually had my own desk, I felt so pleased with myself. It was mine for all the year and I could keep some of my prized items such as old cigarette packets found in the street, a ball of string and well picked but now dead flowers in its wooden frame. Mother could not get at it and I thought I was the only one to know what secrets lay beneath the worn walnut lid. It was MY desk!

On regular occasions the teachers would remove themselves from their high office parked to the right of the blackboard known as their desk. They would walk up and down the rows to observe from their great height any difficulties in the work or sort out any misdemeanours.

My Troubles in the Infants

Times tables were said out loud by the class, route fashion, as teacher walked around tapping the beat with a wooden ruler on the desk as they passed. Like eagles hovering and then swooping on their prey, looking for trouble, more often than not that trouble was me!

Throughout my formal educational life I was prone to these educational birds of prey and their lightning attacks, a lame rabbit stuck on the side of an open mountainside. Each eagle had different methods of attack, some picked me up, often by the ear, and dragged me to the front for a reprimand. Others had the 'I'm too important to waste my time with you but your worthy of me hitting you on the back of your head with my ruler and throwing a quick negative one liner at you' approach.

You see I brought a bag full of detriments with me just to ensure I was singled out before I could be trained to read and write. This bag of detriments was full of ginger hair, a temper to match, freckles, a face only a mother could love and hyperactivity. I'm convinced I had ADHD well before it was popular and had been thought about. That apart I then discovered the worst educational sin of all; being LEFT HANDED! Now, who but his mother could love this devil's child? The 'but' is that they not know that even my own mother hated me?

"Christopher Stewart, we don't write with our left hands here at Moorside," my very first teacher scolded me. What? I just picked up a pencil as expected with a hand, the one that seemed so natural. It was a wrong bordering on evil! Something I did without a pre-thought went totally against the educational establishment I attended. How often was that theme of being deemed so different to re-occur in my struggle to grow into a real human being? My very nature and makeup was in question by those who had the authority to know better and they also had the authority to change me, with whatever methods they decided upon.

I remember I was promptly hauled out to her desk and told to write my lines and letters with my right hand. The control just was not there; this was so against my nature and wrong I thought. Pulling the pencil gave me no more articulation on the paper than any of my preschool scratching by pushing with my left hand. In fact my right arm felt stiff and unable to convert those letters I held in my head as my name into graphite lines that the rest of the world would understand. Should I hold my right hand with my left hand I thought?

I remember such a feeling of helplessness and being so ashamed, in front of the whole class. Tears began to run down my cheeks, silently I thought of words to say about how I was feeling and to correct my dilemma but somehow knew the power of her prejudgment was too strong for me to sway. Any offer of reason would have been an excuse for my sin of wanting to write with my left hand. Frankly, in her eyes, I was not able to write; such a basic task upon which the whole of learning and creativity, even civilisation itself, was built and founded. I was unable to grasp this foundational concept for her. To me I was being ridiculed for being me, like being stripped naked and then poked fun at for having my body.

Her thoughts must have been different, so different to mine. She could save me from this evil, must have ran through her mind. How foolish was I to think that I had lost all hope at such an early age when a tried and trusted correction concept was so readily at hand. No pun intended!

Following all her learning and knowledge of this, my predicament, she knew she could cure me! Not quite knowing what or how she was to do it I was to be excluded from my peers and taken next to that hallowed ground, her desk. I dried my tears and stood while she lent down and pulled from her wooden draw three elastic bands.

"Now Christopher, this is just going to help you write with your proper hand," was her explanation. She gently bound together the fingers of my left hand with the elastic. It was not tight, neither was the little cloth she covered the band with.

The pain was not physical, the pain was the deep traumatic shock a four-year-old felt when his world was rocked and ridiculed by the all-powerful people around him. Is there part of my body unacceptable to the world? Could she just not let me be me! Could she not understand I came to school only to escape the troubles and fears I had at home? School was to be a respite, my holiday on a daily basis away from mother. Why should my failings, so consistently drummed into me at home, surface here, in a real society? I trundled back to my place, watched by all the other children. Perhaps they had not seen anyone with such a curse before.

My disability was to influence nearly all my outcomes of life, especially in educational circles. It was to direct my behaviours and fuel a reputation that preceded me wherever I was to go. This was only the start; because for me it would only get worse. I had a curse. It is the curse of Dyslexia. I had it well before it became researched and given a name. How it manifested itself was the same then as it does today for me. It was as complex as my thinking patterns and yet made me look so simple. It was a curse that covered any intellect with the inadequacies that I have around using the normal methods of communication. It was and still is a curse I carry. No cure, then or now, just techniques to mask it or go around it making me look normal. Any blessings from the disability such as artistic talent were not allowed to surface in such a tight regime used to deliver education in those days.

The unsuccessful hand tying technique was dropped after a while. My writing must have been so much worse and difficult to read. I just struggled so much and the teacher eventually just gave in to my nature. I was allowed to write with my left hand. I had won a small success but only went from worse back to bad again with any form of writing.

Time wasted in those early days trying to correct my natural flow also made me get behind the others in my class. Behind in several basics that I was never to learn or catch up with, rudiments in communication you may have already forgotten or subconsciously used without even a blink of thought about. Detriments that, to this day, still crop up as inadequacies which could have been eradicated by those in control of my learning back then. If only they had known?

I had the curse. It is the curse of not understanding or remembering long verbal instructions first time around, not understanding the letters and how they made words. It is the curse of not comprehending logical sequences, not being able to read the black lines on pages that made words. It is the curse of d's and b's that were forever the wrong way around, a concentration span that lasted only to the end of the first sentence of any instruction.

A curse of putting vowels all over the place in long words completely misspelling them. It is the curse of having a hand that would not form the neat lines and squiggles that constituted legible writing. Not bad for a pencil pusher not puller.

I now wonder how I would have fared at school today as education has hopefully educated itself about this condition. I may not have had this 'rich' story to tell if I was born a generation or two later, or maybe just watered it down to my family's misgivings.

There was also another in built curse I had during my time at Moorside. It was the curse of following, but being nothing like, my older brother Alan. He previously passed through each class that I entered gaining top marks for being clever. At times I was mistakenly called Alan by teaching staff as I followed his footsteps four years behind. In correction the negative comparisons were then thrust upon me as I struggled to comprehend and keep up. Teachers were forever giving me explanations of how he was so good at reading this or writing that. This never enhanced the understanding of my inadequacies. It only sought to embed in me a jealousy of him who was so right all the time, my brother Alan.

I was to gain more short-lived negative fame whilst I progressed through Moorside as a cheeky, disruptive and over active little boy with a crop of ginger hair, a face splattered in freckles, forever in trouble, and thick! Thick! Boy did those controlling the classrooms, the teachers, often aimed that educational term, 'thick', at me!

They had total power within the classroom, were above reproach in their distribution of praise and punishment and well practiced in how to deliver both resources. You see one must remember the politically correct hierarchy of social workers and educational psychologists had not yet invented the term dyslexia. Kids like me then were just labelled, thick and naughty.

Thick because I could not follow the pace of the chalk and talk method of delivering education. Naughty, because after many times of trying to follow and learn I gradually gave up. I had decided my own sideshow would be better to relieve the fact that others were holding on and keeping up with the information delivered in such beautiful chalk scripts on the blackboard. So a little self entertainment of flicking paper balls or talking to whoever was next to me would be far more self stimulating than being lost in the words talked at me or having to try to read.

My continually getting caught malingering during my

formal education only compounded the negative thoughts of those wizened educationalists. Year upon year teacher after teacher must have been convinced I was a dead loss, a hopeless case, a trouble maker and the sooner I was out of their class the better.

I now have the depth of understanding through my work as to what happens in school staff rooms. Chatter about the naughty boy, passing the name on to the next year's educationalist as 'one to watch' is a standard procedure. It's done everywhere. I know, I've seen it long after I was a victim of it. In fact if the truth was known I've done it myself as a FE lecturer, how crass of me!

What type of information is useful to know? Daydreamers, toilet wanting whenever he feels like and used as an excuse, perpetual homework looser, just downright naughty. Lazy through and through. Got a brain but just does not use it. He's a sly one is that, watch him and of course the classic: Don't let him get away with anything, go in hard first and show him who's boss!

Daydreaming was my other classic action for maintaining any sanity I had. A most useful escape whenever I lost the plot of a lesson or was still struggling to understand the first line of the wordy conversation teacher was having with the class.

I had perfected the time worn practice of an unreality activity, daydreaming. I could transfer myself into any part of the world at any given time in the flash of an eye lid without moving from the classroom. The times I was Ivanhoe, that brave knight, fighting to save what is right and just in this world. I would gallop in my head across vast fields of medieval armour clad troops slashing out with my ruler, no, sorry, sword to rescue a family trapped in the clutches of their evil landlord.

Robin Hood also loomed large in my pretences. Robin was a hero known for righting wrongs and lived in the woods. Such a heaven for me and a life style I always wanted to relate to. Often I would ride in my head effortlessly on an elephant, through the Indian jungles hunting for tigers. I could even sit in a space ship, tethered in the school playground awaiting the control centre, back in the headmaster's office, to thrust me high into space. My wave back to earth was one I mirrored from the pictures eagerly scanned into my brain by me in the one space book I possessed. William Tell was another person who I mirrored, gaining the love of the villagers when I sliced the apple on top of my son's head.

I could not fully follow the stories well in books but gained far greater insights from reading every dot on each picture in the reading matter I handled. The one line clips under any picture were enough fuel for me to understand exactly how to get to India, back into medieval times or even to the moon.

"Whack!" The palm of the teacher or their wooden ruler cracking across my head instantly halted any travels I was having in my imagination. "What did I just say?" or "Christopher Stewart, are you listening to me?" would be the verbal interjection enhancing the return to the dreaded here and now.

My Troubles in the Infants

Funny how such simple catchphrases kept repeating themselves, just like history and they would continue to rule elements of my life for many years to come.

My excuses were always lame and often I was vilified in front of the class to end up facing the wall next to the teachers desk or outside on the corridor, face against the wall counting the air holes in each solid red Accrington brick that held the school together.

A brick I counted regularly had nearly twenty five air holes in it. I often wondered how the school ever managed to stand up with so many faulty bricks in its construction. Perhaps one day it would fall down, and then I could go rescue some of the other pupils and go home a hero! Never to be hit, smacked or ridiculed ever again and able to live in the woods, sleep under the stars in that natural environment I loved so much.

No such luck, I just had to stand there, counting the air holes. I suppose it did give me more time to take adventures in my head. I could go walking down the earthen paths in Wardley woods, watching rabbits, and then lie covered with leaves outside the badgers pit awaiting the majestic appearance of the king of the woodland. There were times in the holidays when I would build small wooden huts from twigs and cover them with smaller branches and leaves. I was a Hobbit house builder before the films made them popular. Of course the books were around in my childhood but guess what? I never read them.

Stood against the wall of the corridor I could smell the leaf mould compost covering the ground in those old deciduous woodlands whilst I was in isolation from education. It was a far cry from the so called punishment I was supposed to endure whilst I stood there.

On reflection I guess isolation tactics were not for my benefit but those left within the classroom. I was delivered or given up by the teachers for the education and example of the other pupils. I was sacrificially sent out so that others could get on with their lesson. I was the one sent out as an example of what would happen if you were naughty. Ridiculed and segregated because I was always ready to commit a behavioural disturbance. I, Christopher Stewart, was an easy target.

In that excluded world on the corridor it was also impossible for me to disrupt the class and I left them to learn by rote whatever was included in the day's building block of knowledge for their life's education. Me? I just learnt the intimacies of another real building block supporting the walls of this educational establishment. Education? I was rapidly losing any foundations and support needed to encourage overcoming my difficulties. No basics were drilled in especially in English, right up to today I still don't know what a pronoun or adjective does! Frankly I have got this far without knowing what either is but then again, is that a wise statement?

All this isolation was a double edged curse for me. Self-confidence and belief in myself as an adequate human being was constantly being diminished, added to this was the behaviours enforced by both physical control and ridicule. Unknowingly both mother and school were driving a side each on the duel carriageway towards what should have been my psychological destruction.

Unfortunately as a young person of primary years I was not wise enough to understand my disability or question the authority misplaced in others controlling my life. I had to believe what I was told and I just saw that I was cursed, evil and wicked; as mother retorted so often. 'I had the Devil in me'.

It was to take many years before I would realise, understand, and then dismantle the misconceptions that marred and broke my early years. It would also take working in the most supportive and therapeutic educational environment I would ever know to do it. It took another educational establishment, Lancaster Specialist College, to dismantle the wrongdoings of formal learning in my past and release me to be the person I am today.

I also needed the love of a wonderful, caring woman as the catalyst to complete the self healing process. Both these work and home lives had to be caressed therapeutically at the same time for me to really unearth my demons and expose them to the light.

Letting these negatives shrivel up and die in the warmth has taken so long and is a lifetime away from standing on the school corridor or trying to write with those scratchy ink nibs on the thin wooden pens. Pen nibs in those days were designed to be pulled across the paper to create wonderful script writing. I just pushed them into the paper to give the page an overall look of being spasmodically splattered from on high with India's darkest blue. The comment in red at the bottom of one classic essay was.

"Please don't let your pet spider come to school again." Sarcasm lost on me but probably self gratifying for the writer at the time.

● ● ●

"My body might not always do everything I want,
BUT I am not disabled!"

Beth Moulam

11

My First Love

Schooling in the Infants was not all bad for me. I did have some highlights good enough to share with those who want to listen.

We had in those days a particular way in the play ground of collecting other children to play with. It did not have a name as I know it but went similar to this. A small number of boys would decide to play a group game such as football or girls say cats and cradles. To see if others in the yard wanted to play they would link arms and march around the playing area shouting their intentions in a chant such as "Who's playing football?" or "Who's playing Rawhide?" Any of the interested children could then link arms to the end and be a part of the picking system when it broke up and teams were decided.

Guess who was always picked last to the football team

and more than ever ended up being the goalie, a position all the others never wanted to play? Little old Christopher Stewart, that's who. Football was all about scoring goals at that tender age and not standing between two jackets or pullovers slung on the playground floor, just to graze one's knees on the tarmac when diving to save the shots.

It was in one of these social outside plays that I managed to engage a certain Yvonne Cassidy. She was a real peach of a girl, same age as me, about five or six at the time. Yvonne had blond hair that was always in pigtails and a soft smile with white teeth that always shone at me. I asked her quite boldly if I could play skipping with her and to my great delight she said yes. Wow, a real girl wanting to play with me. I never questioned it at the time but with hindsight it could have been in sympathy, who knows? We skipped till the bell went to signal end of play time and I went into classes.

She was of the same year as me, went to the same school as me, was even in the same class as me but was so different to me. She smelled different and made me look at her differently. She was often in my thoughts and never refused when I wanted to play with her, albeit it on her terms, never Footy or Cowboys and Indians.

One day before school started and the early birds were playing she rushed over to me with a small envelope in her hand. It was pink and I opened it with a rush. I tried to read the script writing but before I made another fool of myself she blurted out. "It's an invitation to my birthday party, can you come?"

"Yes," I instantly replied, "I'll come!" She skipped off in a happy state that only a child can have when the world is hers.

I then did a reality check and thought of what Mother would say. All day it was kept in my trouser pocket and I had to continually pull it out to look at to ensure it was real and was not another figment of my imagination. Was it really for me? I smelt it again and again. It must have smelt like the sweetest French perfume. It smelt of her!

I rushed to the gate at the end of the school day to hand mother the now crumpled envelope.

"Yvonne has asked me to go to her birthday party," I blurted out. We never had parties to celebrate our birthdays at home, it would have been too much pressure and hassle for mother and for Christopher Stewart to get an invite to others was almost as rare. Mother looked at the invitation inside the creased envelope and smiled at me. She had seen Yvonne before and talked to her when Yvonne accompanied me to the gates sometimes at the end of the school day.

Now I can only presume she told others that I had a girl friend as parents do with an element of humour when their immature child has such a platonic friendship.

"Has she told you where she lives?" Mother still had the smile on her face.

"No but can I still go? It's on a Saturday."

The reason for Mother's wry smiles was that Yvonne, lived in a very grand detached Edwardian house on Monton Green overlooking the golf course, homes where only the rich and elegant lived locally! Evidently her father was a publisher and was a top earner in his day. All this was lost on Yvonne who was sugar sweet and honestly innocent of the world at large. The fact that she had befriended me was certification of that fact.

I went to the party. I remember feeling rather out of place, especially after the threats mother gave me before hand if I did anything wrong. Yvonne kept our friendship up after this but for me it was never the same. I must have realised that her upbringing was so far removed from mine and I just did not fit into her opulence. I can remember it frightened me a little feeling so far behind in manners, money and elegance.

She left our primary school and I'm sure she went to a private one to better her education. I never forgot her and her beautiful smell, it was the first time I had ever had a loving and kind relationship with a female. Years later when I was in my late twenties we met up again by chance and instantly she recognised me. Well who could forget the freckle faced ginger nut from school with such an outgoing personality? She was still as sweet and said a wonderful thing to me then. "Do you know," she quietly asked me, "that you were the very first boy to ever kiss me on the lips and I remember it so well."

"Oops!" What an impression I must have made! We never kept in touch but, it was a good thing at the time, unfortunately by the age of eight I must have just grown out of it!

Another girl that was to impress her name and life into

my mind at that age but for totally different reasons was Margaret Dutton. Poor Margaret, she was to hold a very special place for me, if only I could have somehow told her.

We started that fateful day in school gathering in the classroom being told that we were to have a special assembly in the hall before lessons began. All the infants piled in and the head teacher was in front. We were drilled into moving into the spacious room in silence and the teaching staff stood alongside their allocated form for that year. It was a controlling position so they could see along the row to who was making noises or trying to talk.

Today the teachers seemed extra controlling and we all soon suspected something different had happened. A hymn was sung from the large sheets that were flipped over and hung high on the wall at the front. Then the head stood up and spoke in very solemn tones. He explained that one of the pupils had been in a very serious accident the previous day, and had died then gone to heaven to be with Jesus and the other angels. That pupil was Margret Dutton.

Her name was mentioned in a hushed tone. She was in my class and at the sound of her name I remember looking along the row for her. No she was not there and the head must be telling the truth. I felt a little numb and we finished the assembly with another hymn and prayers for her and her family. I still did not let the reality of her passing sink in until I went back to the class.

The teacher was conscious of all the facts and understood the gravity of the situation. Apparently Margaret was killed in a house fire at her home. More than that I do not know but cry I did and again I was fortunate that my special friends came to comfort me on several nights since her demise. I was an emotional child, still am as an adult, and always let my feelings show through tears or getting upset for the down trodden or those in pain.

The death of a class mate so young was another blow for me, the stark fact that life could be so short left me upset for Margaret and hurt me in a way I had not been hurt before. I was not upset about my own sad little life this time, now it was very different. The demise of someone else I knew and had played with in the yard had made an impact so deep I can recall it so clearly today many years after the event. The reality of never being able to see her again was one that I won't forget.

Some nights I would go to sleep asking her to look after me and save me a place alongside her if the worst ever happened to me because of Mother. She did not appear to me directly as a special friend but I dreamt of her often after her tragic leaving, both as before her death when a playmate and after it, as an angel.

12

Ringing the Bell

Once and once only did I try to turn the educational system of the infants upside down and fight it from my corner. Well not really, but at that young and tender age it must have been like a David and Goliath scenario. But instead of standing and fighting my cause, I just ran away, although quite spectacularly even if I say so myself.

There was one occasion I tried to correct the wrongs done to me which gave me a valuable lesson in life. Running away is never the answer; it only gives a temporary halt to the difficulties, which tend to catch up with you sooner or later. Just like lies, they always have a nasty habit of biting you in the bum later, usually when you least expect it.

I vividly remember the afternoon in the infants when I temporarily broke free from the curse and released myself for a few hours! I could only have been six or seven but it was another day I was to suffer ridicule yet again. I had decided to take a brave and decisive action that would tar me for the rest of my life in that part of the school!

Once again in class I could not write the words from the board, so finely scripted for me to copy. My hand would not transfer the flowing lines in the order my eyes saw them. My work was a mess. I gave up and began my disruptive behaviour. Today this would have been seen as a sign of my specific educational difficulties but back then I was in immediate trouble with the room's authority.

The rules were simple in those days for corporal punishment. In the infants a ruler or slap at the back of the legs. From the age of about six in the junior's you could be caned on the hand by the class teacher or on the bum by the head teacher. The latter had to be logged in the punishment book.

In the secondary school from 11 upwards you were in the big boy's league. Class teachers could cane or slipper you at will. Crimes that needed the heads intervention meant that you were caned six times on the bum and both the crime and punishment were logged in the punishment book.

How do I know so precisely this list? Well I learn all my information through practical methods, not by reading or talking about the theory. Learning about the punishment regime in my school was no different!

Dragged out to the front, the ruler came down with a ferocious whack against my right hand. To ensure a perfect and painful contact the teacher held my wrist with her hand underneath. Each blow really hurt and I can remember holding my red marked hand, throbbing with pain and trying to quell the sensation by writhing my fingers on my left hand. I cried and cried, not loudly but with whimpers that had to be controlled. As I stood there, in front of my classmates, I felt as diminished and belittled as a child could ever be. I wanted to die. I could not run because I knew the consequences would be far too great.

There was no escape from the corporal punishment inflicted or the psychological punishment that went along with being berated in front of all. I was also to stand and suffer my fate of pain and ridicule by being sent out into the corridor facing the wall.

I was ushered away with another string of ridicule to stand in place facing my bricks. These baked oblongs were at least always neutral to me, never to mock or demise me. I knew them, and they knew me but today I had just been sent to a new low and felt I had to get away. How could I do it? There was never to be an outside incident, a disaster intervening to save me and let me be normal again. I needed to do something myself.

The corridor went the full length of the infant's school. On one side was a continuous line of classrooms, only broken by the dining/assembly hall/gym in the middle. On the other side were two grassed square areas open to the elements, interrupted only by the head and deputy head's office slap bang in the middle.

Outside the deputy head's office was The Bell. This was no ordinary bell. It had control and influence over the whole infant school, its staff and pupils. It was a large push button affair about three feet off the floor. It was rung to summon changes of routine in the school day. School timings, coming and goings therefore were all regimented by The Bell, it rang for the start of the school day then at each break and lunch. The final time the bell rang was home time. Such a simple piece of electrical machinery had such a powerful command over the whole of this institution.

That day I was in corridor isolation in the early afternoon, just after lunch. Could I end this awful day of ridicule early, and get home, at least to exchange the pain of here to one of a different kind.

I looked back into the classroom; teacher was busying herself by marking the work of the others at her desk. I looked up and down the corridor, silence and no one around. Quietly with the stealth of a tiger, the bravery of Ivanhoe and the social justice of Robin Hood, I tiptoed towards the bell. Nearer and nearer, my heat pounded.

Little did I realise my actions that day would be so deeply etched into my subconscious. Even now I can still feel the anxiety as I write this line for you. I reached out and with the accuracy of William Tell my index finger rested on the button. It rang loud and clear across the school. Freedom and release beckoned.

Quickly and quietly I ran towards the cloakroom at the far end of the corridor. I grabbed my tatty blue gabardine and school cap from my peg. I ran away from that place, across the yard and out of the gates as fast as a rocket towards home.

Ringing the Bell

Away from the mockery and disbelief that I was not an ordinary little boy. Away from the disbelief that I was bright and intelligent, just unable to transpose my intellect into words and writing understood by the controlling adults around me. I had opened the gates of my dungeon and released myself from hell.

I ran fast into the subway that took me safely under the great highway connecting Manchester and Liverpool. I ran and ran along the great East Lancashire Road cycle path. I stopped gasping for breath. There, in front of me was my field of dreams, the Clough.

Nestled next to the great dual carriageway half way between home and school this old and unused farm's fields were my first outdoor haven of my earliest days. Two streams ran in large gullies either side of the field and both were filled with frogs, toads, and newts amongst the myriad of wildlife. It was a place where I could play and imagine whatever I wanted and be whoever I needed to be to fulfil those dreams. Trees and bushes enabled me to climb and hide, play and imagine, enabled me to escape. Where else was I to spend this parole time before I was to appear at home on time as if normality ruled the day? The Clough was my dream playground.

Unaware of the troubles I had caused behind me I then blissfully played for the rest of the afternoon amongst the streams, building dams, repairing banks, swinging from trees and looking for rat and vole holes. Later, when I noticed other pupils walking home along the side of the Clough, on the cycleway of the East Lancashire Road, I decided it was time for me to go home, as if it was the end of school. A quick wash of my hands in the stream and a dry on the grass of the sunny bank I was ready to appear at home. I was oblivious to the turmoil I had created and walked the half-mile to the semi where I knew mother was.

The justification of my deceit on the extraordinary day was wasted upon mother. Walking into the back room I was instantly aware of the encroaching trauma I was to endure because of my delinquencies.

Mother was sat in her usual angry position. This meant her foot would be tapping the tiles on the hearth of the fireplace and she would be sat with her knees open, hands on her knees and a face like thunder. Sometimes in winter she also poked the burning coals with ferocity that made me think that even the coal fire was afraid of her.

I stood still, rooted to the spot, awaiting her response. "What have you been doing and where the bloody hell have you been?" My incompetent lies were wasted.

"I've just been coming home, along the Clough."

"You bloody liar." With a swipe of her hand sent me across the room, to my knees and crying I crumpled into a corner. "You rang the bell and ran off didn't you?" she reeled out.

How did she know? Could I never be rid of this all-powerful overseer who would make me pay tenfold for each of my misdemeanours? Pay for it I did, I was in for it. To this day I will never know how she knew what I had done but I do remember her idea of punishment dealt so swiftly, sharply and so prolonged.

She reached behind herself to the right hand draw on the old chest of drawers, made during the war. It was a practical cupboard, not pretty, just like the leather belt she pulled from it. I was made to stand on the lino at the edge of the carpet and take my shirt off.

Then in silence, coldly and deliberately she took aim and unleashed the buckle end towards my back. Crack, it went exactly where it was aimed to go. I stood my ground for a second; felt a rush of pain then fell to the floor. "Get up you little swine," she screamed, "I'll make you pay for humiliating me. You little swine, you bastard, why do you always do this to me? I'll have to beat the devil out of you."

This last phrase was used often when I was to really pay for my misdemeanours. She told me on more than a few occasions that I had a devil inside of me and she would beat it out. Strange words for a mother to direct at her young son I know, but I felt she really meant it. Was I the Devil incarnate? Often I would question myself, why me, why her? Did she know I had little friends who would talk to me? They comforted me in times of great pain but were they sent from the devil? Did Mother really have the strength to beat all this out of me? Would the pain of death release me from this hell?

Mother hauled me up again by my ginger mop and started her flurry. The belt worked overtime up and down it whizzed through the air onto my little back and around my legs. I hopped and danced to try to avoid the worst of the pain but it still hurt. Wow, did it hurt!

Seconds felt like hours. I can remember seeing some

blood from my back on the shiny brown lino. She must have broken the skin.

"I'm so sorry I did not mean to do it, I'll never do it again, ever," I cried, I sobbed and really did not want to have this happen to me again.

In hindsight was I really sorry for the evil action or just the punishment I was being subject to. Each frail apology of mine only brought more ferociousness, as if relighting her anger. I cried and wept tears in the midst of the pain, tears of sorrow for myself.

"The Devil!" she cried, "I'll beat the Devil out of you!"

I never knew when the torrent would end when on the receiving end of her rage and resentment. She stopped her physical reprimand, paused for breath then started what the three of us siblings called 'nagging'.

She hurled a torrent of abuse at me. Mother went on and on, and on. I don't just mean for a while, she could nag us for five or six hours at a time. Later in my childhood I was to endure more of these marathon sessions but this time my physical endurance seemed to limit the verbal torrent to about an hour.

She was so angry, very angry. No time now to escape into my fantasies or talk to my little friends in the cupboard or under my bed. I had to concentrate, listening to give the right answers and awaiting the spasmodic flash of the buckle as it came towards my body as if to reassert her physical control. Although it was teatime, around five o'clock, I was sent to bed with only my aching, battered and bleeding body and my pain to comfort me.

Ringing the Bell

This was to be another night that I talked in my head to the imaginary bird in the imaginary cage that I always had sat at the foot of my half of the bed. Real to me. I could always talk to it as a friend, knowing it would never strike, swear at or ridicule me. Asking it questions about my self worth and sanity. Such as: Why did I get this beating? Was I really as wicked and evil as I was told? Silly bird never gave me the answers I wanted or made my world right. Still I never gave up on it, especially when my heart bled and my room was viewed through my watery eyes. My special friends were eventually to take over the role my bird held and they would become more real to me than ever.

13

My Little Friends

I distinctly remember that my name was called from under the bed. Yes I had, on several occasions, especially when the beatings were given in their extreme, been called by some little friends. They came to me quite spontaneously, always when life for me was dark and I felt scared and all alone in a cruel world.

I never had to call them, they just came. They seemed to know me and the turmoil my little mind was in. I never needed to cry out to them, they just came. Over the times they came I remember about three or four different ones but they were all dressed the same, apart from the old man.

Each child was pale faced with large eyes; they wore a white smock like garment and spoke softly all knowing my name. Sometimes they were under my bed, around my age but almost doll size so they fitted upright in the small space.

At the time I never doubted their existence or questioned what they said. Neither was it in my mind or heart to question where they came from, just that they knew me, were always gentle and kind to me and gave me great comfort. Perhaps if I started to question or contradict them they would disappear forever, never to give me the comfort I so longingly needed.

They started to appear to me when I was about four or five and left when I was aged around ten or eleven. My little friends, boys and girls in old fashioned white smocks stood there under the bed and talking and smiling at me. Told me it will all go away they did and I'll be better one day. Did I believe them? I think so at the time, but when they faded I went back into my living hell again, brutally bullied by the one person who should have been my saviour.

One of these 'friends' would appear in the airing cupboard another one sat on the bed next to me. I even had a young girl about my age once walk with me on the way home when I knew I was getting into trouble. Why did they love and care for me? Why did they even want to talk to me? Who were they? Where did they come from? I never asked them at the time nor wanted to know. Comfort and kindness was always their core aim to me.

That was the general gist of their soft conversations except for one day. This particular day, the day I rang the bell and ran away. "Do you want to join me?" she asked. She just stood there with her arms slightly outstretched, smiling with soft lips and sad eyes. I can't think of what I replied but I thought long and hard about what she had said.

Was it simply my imagination taking me to a place where I really wanted to be, out of my world and into another? Taking me far away from Mother and this sad lonely life I had. I'm really not sure if she said those exact words but today I still recall a soft voice asking such a possible life changing question.

I took my special friends for given when they appeared and relied upon them heavily in times of distress. Best kept to myself I thought at the time, don't want anyone to get rid of them for me do I? And those outside of my world would if I told them about my little friends. I was always in enough trouble and just kept them hidden. They were my secret from the rest of the world and I kept this secret hidden for over half a century.

They were the little people I could play with and talk to. They blessed me with a childlike sanity that my other imaginary items did not do and were the most comforting aspects in my life in the darkest times. How could I not love them? I had to keep them to myself, a secret I would never break.

On a very few occasions I was not sure if I was asleep dreaming or not but a kindly old man in a First World War uniform would peer over my bed and, without breathing a word, smile and then seem to fade into the darkness of my room when I tried to contact or talk to him. Who was he? Why was he so real? Why did he come to look at me? I was always left puzzled but never scared.

In retrospect it was spooky and not normal for one so young but at the time it was so comforting and warm. Well who's to say what's normal in such a turbulent infancy? The make believe animals and tins of paint of mine were acceptable to other people but these special friends were different, perhaps they were really real!

The possible answer came to me when I was nearing the latter part of my life. Remarried and happy with every day the Lord gave me I quite sceptically supported my wife on a visit to a medium in Lancaster. She had the desire to go, having spent her childhood with her mother who frequently visited a Spiritualist church. It seemed natural to my wife but she did not have a labyrinth of past activities that may disturb or unsettle her as I did.

On that day I just went along to support really, for no other motive, no quest to lay spirits to rest so to speak. It was held in an ordinary semi detached, very nicely furnished; bright and not too cluttered perched on a hill with fantastic views over Lancaster and Morecambe bay.

I sat in the front room, silent for the most time and took my turn after my dear wife had been 'done'. The medium was a very pleasant woman who explained she had lost her sister in tragic circumstances a few years previously and began then to realise she had a gift to 'contact the other side'. I just let her sit alongside me and, go off on one, into a trance like state whilst I thought, "It's an easy way to earn £20.00!"

Initially she started to breathe in a heavy way then

took some sharp intakes of breath. She began to tell me of people in my past and things she should and could never have known about.

My estranged son was mentioned by name, she said he will eventually get back in touch. Impossible at the present time I thought. An uncle and others from the family were revealed to me by initial or name. She then said I had been visited as a child by child spirits that played with me!

It stunned me to hear a complete stranger tell me about things she had no knowledge about. I had never told anyone about the 'friends' who used to visit me. The medium explained that she was only an interpreter for the 'other side' and what she said was being told to her by people in the spirit world. She said I had seen spirits when I was a child, and they played with me and talked to me. She was right, these friends must have been just that.

I sat there half mesmerised, half terrorised, not knowing what to say or do. Fight or flight kicked in again but I just sat and listened spellbound to the words formed from beyond. I suppose before I actually got there I sneakily thought if it was going to be true about contact from the dead then I hope my dad would get in touch. It was not to be. Dramatically for me it was Mother.

"Your Mother is here," she said. You just can't imagine what I was feeling. I just drained and my guts turned over and over. I then felt an overwhelming urge to get up and leave the room, not wishing to face one so powerful and evil to me. Was she really here? Could I tell her what I truly though of her? Of how she threw away the innocence of my childhood and replaced it with fear, self doubt and pain.

The medium lent over towards me and said,"She says that there is no malice but only forgiveness in the Spirit world." Why would the medium say these things to me? She knew nothing about my childhood. Was I to believe her? Then the next sentence threw me even further into a confused state. "Your mother is asking about your diary."

Well where did that come from? I never kept a diary, was never self-disciplined enough and besides it entailed writing. "Diary. I don't have a diary and have never kept one, I don't know what she means," I replied, almost in tones to ridicule the message giver.

Once these words left my lips I wished I had never said them. This book, my book, the one about me, was this book what she meant as my diary? Did Mother mean my writing about her and her ways? Mother must have known what I had written so far and she was asking me about it.

I now have to take some time to reiterate that this is not a novel scripted from an author's imagination, far from it. Both my wife and the medium can verify what was said in that room. Mother was asking me, through the medium, about this book. Was I to believe it? Well I have no other answer for the knowledge the medium had of me. What was I to say?

Writing about someone who was long dead was far easier on my soul than having her there in the room, asking about my thoughts transferred into script for the world to see. Was this to stop me, did she really mean that from the grave she still had a power over me that she could continue into my adulthood? "All is forgiven in the Spirit world," the medium said again, as if to ensure that the words entered into my whirring thoughts and stayed in the memory.

Having had no real comprehension of the written word as a child I have crafted some coping skills to compensate for my many educational failings. Dyslexics do this I am informed. Using my mouth as an oral projector of words without contemplation beforehand has been, on occasions, a saviour, as well as causing me to crawl under the nearest stone when I got it wrong.

I used this 'mouth before brain' skill without thought of the consequences. "What does she want me to do about the book?" I asked the medium, still not wishing to fully recognise that Mother was there.

"Publish," the reply instantly came from the lady sat next to me with her eyes closed, head held slightly back and mouth open. I felt a smile inside me, a warm self satisfied feeling only occasionally felt in a long and incident filled life.

My book was the only thing I had done to counter all the pain of my Dyslexic childhood. I would be able to give others an understanding of me by using the channels of communication, the same written words, that initially failed me and made the world see me as an idiot. I would have conquered the devil in my life and Mother, yes Mother, was telling me from beyond that I was to do it. No feelings of remorse or forgiveness came over me, just a quiet satisfaction that there might come a conclusion to this through my conquering of the written word.

As a practicing Christian I still don't partake in the whole spiritualist thing but I can't help believing that I was visited when a child and it was not just figments of my imagination that helped me through those evil times. I guess the answer will only truly be revealed when I cross to the other side! I have prayed to my Lord since then for answers to these questions. His answer is yet to be revealed but I wait patiently.

The night of Ringing the Bell had been yet another night I slid into sleep hugging a pillow wet from my tears and feeling demonised for being myself. The little friends had gone and I was left alone again. My childhood was littered with too many nights such as these.

If I was to believe the propaganda so harshly dealt to me I would have ended it all myself. Was the troubled birth I had really worth surviving only, to endure the life I was trying to live? Would such a worthless troublemaker be missed on this God's earth? No, I was not worthy of being missed. "Just let me go, not wake up tomorrow," I cried softly to the Man upstairs. I endured many such horrors as a young child but it was not until my mid teenage years that I really tried to exit this world by my own accord.

As a small child, how was I to break this cycle of hurt, fear, pain and worthlessness inflicted upon me by those who controlled my life? I could not escape except into my own world of fantasy and make-believe. Once old enough to play out on my own then I would find sweet respite in places of nature, The Clough and the Indoo's behind the

Town Hall and Wardley Woods were open places within a short walk or cycle ride of home.

Until I was allowed out so far I was to remain a child locked into a world of violence and mental instability, a cruelty known about by neighbours but who would not interfere to rescue me. It was just not the thing to do in those days.

Incidentally when I did get back to school I was to spend the first day back stood outside the deputy heads office, facing the wall on show to all for my misdemeanours. I was caned and it was put in the book. I was told in no uncertain terms what would happen to me at school if I was to attempt such naughtiness ever again. Little did they know it was an idle threat in comparison to the punishment dealt out by my mother's own hands? Her methods of correction were known only to those in the house. Our neighbours must have suspected but nothing was ever done.

14

Winter and the Grey Snow Falling

Although I preferred summer as a small child I revelled in the extremities winter brought in the weather. Those days were full of the smog, rain and snow affected by the vast industrial area I grew up in.

Trafford Park was only across the Ship Canal and I could see its great industrial chimneys from various vantage points on the upper reaches of Partington Lane in Swinton. The Clean Air Act did create a cleaner living environment and I was all the better for it, but the previously chronic atmosphere did hold its own quirky pleasures for me.

The Park, as we called Trafford Park, was the immense throbbing industrial heart of Manchester, the power house of its industry. The wind invariably blew a south westerly from the Atlantic across south Lancashire towards Salford, catching the putrid fumes and exhausts from countless industrial chimneys and fires and held on to it long enough to carry it towards the dirty old town. Invariably it would relinquish some of its chemical particles as it floated overhead. This made the privets and windows dirty enough to require cleaning and shaking on a regular basis. We used to clean the outside of the windows with newspaper many an evening just after it had gone dark, stood on a chair, removing the grime. I could also taste the air in those days, a dry chemically taste which had a smell I have never smelt again since. Coughs and colds were rampant as were other long term bronchial illnesses that made most adults wheeze and splutter in the depths of winter.

When it did snow it was never a Christmas card white landscape but a grey tinge that covered the roads and houses. The smog was another element that altered after the Clean Air Act came into force. Previously smog covered the town on a regular basis on winter's short days. It was a collection of fog, dirt and chemicals. It was thick and putrid and left a sticky film covering everything outside.

One dark winter's eve I happened to go along Worsley Road to Saint Stephen's church hall for a Church Lads Brigade night. The fog was so thick I could not tell where the pavement ended and the road started. I had to call on my memory to get me up to the old church hall.

There was always a chill, deadening of sound on these nights. Suddenly I could hear a man's voice and then the dimmed thudding of an old diesel motor. It was a bus trying to negotiate the pea souper. The guard had to walk very slowly in front of the bus on the road and direct the driver which way he was to go and warn against any parked cars on the road. The faint lights from the headlights were of little use against such a thick still cloud of moisture and chemicals.

Deadly as it was for many folks I loved it. This tangible cloud enabled me to travel to another planet where it was full of gas and my balaclava was the only protection from the poison like a Spaceman's helmet. With my woollen protector as my mask I would encounter Martians in doorways and twelve headed snakes appearing from every other grid. I slaughtered more earth threatening creatures that stalked the streets of Swinton on nights like those than any other night. In this weather no one could see me and laugh at such a child's imagination. It was an eerie playground for me to imagine in but one I took full advantage of when it appeared.

There was also the annual fall of snow in November or early December that heralded the nearness of Christmas. I vividly recall looking out of the cold front room window one evening, head under the curtains and nose pressed against the cold window pane. Mother was in the back room with the fire knitting one of our many hand crafted jumpers or string vests.

I could see the dim street light in the drive which was almost parallel with our front garden. It highlighted the flurry of soft tinged snow that was falling constantly. No cars, no people walking up the drive just snow, the light, the rest of the drive in darkness, and me. It looked like bliss and sounded so silent, as silent as the night the carol had us believe that Jesus was born.

I watched the snow for ages and ages until I was numb with cold in the little unheated room. I would occasionally look skyward just to see if there was really a sleigh going about its business, preparing for Christmas Eve. That night I saw a faint flashing red light in the sky move above the houses across the drive. There was a magic about it all.

I really did believe and I knew deep inside I had goodness inside me screaming to get out. I pleaded to the man I thought was riding the sleigh I thought I saw that winter's night. "Don't believe what the adults say about me and miss me out. Please believe me, oh please, please believe me, wherever you are. I am good and just want to live a normal life," I believed I was talking to the Father of Christmas and he could weave his magic to make things better for me.

Another particular day in the winter I remember, which was also a national tragedy, was Feb 7th 1958. How can I be so precise about the date when I can not remember what was said to me five minutes previously? It was the time of a national tragedy. I would be six at the time.

Coming up our Drive it was dark and I could see the women of the street were standing under the lamppost, which was the only light in the drive. They were talking very quietly and I could see they were upset, some crying and the group were reading copies of the Manchester Evening News in the poorly shed light and cold. It was the day after the Munich Air disaster in which seven of the

Manchester United team died returning from a European Cup game. It was a Salford tragedy as well as a national one for two of the team were local lads.

This scene is etched in my mind along with all the others but especially as my father had previously taken me on occasions to Old Trafford to watch the Red Devils play. Who they played or the score I cannot remember but for such a young boy to be in a crowd of sixty thousand plus was an occasion I recall with some relish and detail.

Dad was born and brought up in Salford and it was just as natural for those in the dirty old town to go to over the Ship Canal into Trafford and watch Manchester United for their Saturday afternoon entertainment as it was to get drunk and eat fish and chips on a Friday night.

As soon as I was old enough dad would take me to see his beloved Reds and I was enraptured by the immense size and stimulation of the occasion. I can still see clearly from where I stood at the front against a small wooden fence, the team mascot walking around the edge of the pitch before the game in his red and white top hat and tails.

Every other youngster seemed to have a wooden rattle which they turned around above their heads at any exciting part of the play or when their team entered the arena like gladiators. The noise made when the teams came out and later, when the home team slotted the ball into the back of the net, was deafening. I saw little of the game because I was so small but the sensory experience I experienced was absorbed into my history. The feel of being in a crowd of so many humans, the smell of the pies and overflowing toilets etched into my memory bank. I remember my excitement lived long after the final whistle and Dad must have thought he had created another lifelong Red's fan.

How would Dad have coped today if he knew I had defected to the blue side of town? Manchester City now has my allegiance. "Why change colours half way through life?" he may have asked me.

I really became disillusioned with the money and power games going into Old Trafford many years ago. Manchester United wielded huge power and influence on the game as they grew into the richest football team in the world. I kept my feet firmly on the floor and politically the thought of money bringing such influence is far from my social and Christian ethics. The richer they got the further away from my heart they went.

Surely Sir Matt Busby would be turning in his grave if he knew the shenanigans going on today and the money and bungs sloshing around the clubs. I was told he used to ask his players at the end of the game two things:

"Had they enjoyed themselves and had they played their best?" Today results and league positions are to dependent on how much money the team has. If you lost in my youth pride was at stake and Denis Law was paid only around £75.00 each week! Today at Old Trafford if they lose people look up how much money was wiped off their shares. Defiantly not football to me, I value an even playing field and the game played for it own sake.

Man City needed my support in their 30 odd years of

drought and who else puts a smile on the faces of real football fans when you mention that you follow them?

Manchester United play in the largest team stadium in the country. It is built to hold as many fee-paying fans as possible to make as much money each home game as possible. An income of three million pounds gross, at the last count, for each home game to a club so deep in debt, surly the figures do not balance?

Spectators in the uppermost tiers are so far away they cannot see nor have any contact with the players on the pitch so far below them. They must also win a trophy every season. If not then their season has been disastrous. I do not relate to that as being the 'people's game'.

Today City play in their new stadium, which is owned by Manchester City Council. It's proudly boasts to being the biggest council house in Manchester! To string several wins together (two!) sends their fans into a tizzy of excitement and dreams of beating the local rags twice a season is stuff City fans live off. I too can live with that.

How things have changed from the days when I first was taken to watch the beautiful game and when those local lads died for the club they loved.

How things have changed since I first wrote these words? Now City is the richest club in the world, owned by one of the richest men in the world. With all that wealth comes an air of expectancy. Saying that, when I do go to the City games looking around at the spectators they are the type of people who always supported this, their local team, all locals to the Manchester area. Their accent and humour is still undeniably working class and from within the vicinity of old South East Lancashire. Not so just outside the town to Trafford (Incidentally not in Manchester) where the rest of the crowd is made up from oriental tourists, southerners, Irish and Scots!

15

Dad Chucked Out

Dad must have left soon after he took me to watch the football. He had been promoted at the hospital and was to earn a princely sum as a night Charge Nurse. Mother was having none of it. She wanted her husband to be there every night, not working hard to earn the money for the new mortgage, and boy did she let him know in no uncertain terms.

It was enough he went to Ardwick, across Manchester once a week to the Territorial Army barracks. He would also disappear odd weekends on camp and had a fortnight full summer camp every year. Working nights in addition was just not acceptable to her.

Screaming arguments ensued, even worse than before, some violent but often ending with Jim saying: "Right that's it I've had enough I'm off." Initially if it was early enough in the day or at weekend she would retort.

"You can take him with you," the 'him' meaning me! I was a handful, always in trouble, clumsy and breaking pots and falling over furniture and it would have been better for her if I was out of the way. Alan of course always reading and quiet was never ushered away. It would also have meant that Jim had a chaperone. I suppose she was a crafty bitch, just like Dad said.

Eventually, to avoid these flash points, he would return from work at tea time then initiate going out with. "I'm taking Chris out to the pictures with me." Life at that age can be so dictated by such a simple catch phrase. It was the get out clause used to remove ourselves from the fray. Mother would run a torrent of abuse at him as he got my coat and we left just after tea to turn up at one of the three flea pits masquerading as cinemas in Swinton.

Yet I was to enter another magical world as we watched The Wizard of OZ, Bridge over the River Kwai, and Holiday Inn. Old Yella and Greyfrier's Bobby would always make me push back into the hard cinema seat so no one could see the streams of tears rolling down my face.

I never saw my dad laugh much but he did when I hid behind the seat in front the first time the green faced witch appeared in the Wizard of Oz. She still has a chilling effect today, some 70 years after she first appeared.

My mother I hated, but this evil witch scared me in a different way. I recognised the evil in her and had developed a third sense that she was wicked to the extreme.

The films were often seen more than once. I could go

to school with the moments of excitement or horror from the big screen flashing around my memory box. I was word perfect at such a young age on parts of so many classic 50's movies. Shame I always had to return home to rush upstairs to bed and leave them two continuing to argue until dad came to bed in our room.

Another place I was taken to as a nipper was his army barracks. Dad never really left the Army. He was in the Territorial Army before WW2 started, which meant he was called up in 1939 as part of the BEF in France. When I got to know him again towards the end of his life he spoke little of what he experienced during the war. I gleaned snippets from him and his sisters padded them out for me with what he really went through.

His army career as a medic took him first retreating across France to Dunkirk where he escaped the blood bath of the beaches just wearing his underclothes and towels. He had to shed his heavy army uniform to stand in the water for hours before being picked up by one of the fleet of little ships.

Later after some recuperation Dad was shipped off to India to fight in the forgotten war against the Japanese. His six months behind enemy lines with the Chindit's also gave one or two very impressionable stories.

On demob from this 'scrap' he continued his part time life in the TA as a medic gaining rank as Mess Sergeant in his latter days at Ardwick barracks, Manchester. My aunts told me long after he died the day he had to retire from the TA was the beginning of his life going downhill and eventually dying of cancer at 62.

Meanwhile this escape time from mother, in the place he took me to, was again fantastic for such a little boy such as myself and set me off again into a play world of fantasy. At the back of the TA drill hall was a large garage full of trucks, ambulances and Landrovers all in the Army camouflage.

Whilst he was in the mess I would be given free range of this adult play area. Without turning an engine, I toured all the battlefields of the war in my imagination, sitting behind each steering wheel. Whilst making all the noises of a child fighting with pretend guns makes, revving sounds made to take the truck up hill and down a jungle track without even moving a wheel. I swung from the tops of canvas trucks, hid in ambulances and clambered up excessively large four wheel drive twenty two ton field trucks. For me it really was child's pretend play with men's toys.

Dad left Stonegate Drive to live with his sister back in Weaste after literally having his things chucked out by mother. Trauma leaves you with indelible memories. I saw his clothes being thrown through the open front door and outside onto the small grass area called our front garden.

"If you think you can work nights and still be a father and husband then this is what I think of it. Go on, beggar off to bloody Weaste." Any neighbours watching kept a discrete distance behind the curtains but the noise would have been enough to attract their attention. Poor man, we as kids were not embarrassed just scared but I bet he must have been ashamed.

Dad Chucked Out

I knew that day that he was leaving my life. I was to be left defenceless against this woman who would dictate and control my formative years. I remember crying, whether it was for me or for my father I cannot remember but with hindsight it was because of the illness that was to control her whilst she fought keep total control over her children.

Weaste is only the name of a part of Salford where my dad moved to but the word soon became an icon used in our house for all that was bad and evil in the world.

"You don't live in Weaste!" was used whenever I left things out or did something wrong. "Go on get to bloody Weaste then, see if he'll look after you!" was another phrase used, supposedly to send shivers down my spine when I had done wrong.

Mother ran a campaign of hatred using that particular part of the dirty old town as verbal ammunition, so often aimed at me. To a greater extent that was easier than the bullets of humiliation and pain she also used in the name of control.

16

The Weybridge Holiday

You cannot imagine how financially poor we were when Dad left. He sent his money, called 'Maintenance', in cash every Friday by a registered envelope. Mother had the indignity of having to wait for the post man to ring the bell on our front door and she would sign for it.

Dad was very regular with sending it but on the occasional times it was a day late there was all hell on. It would put mother in a foul mood and she had her habit of taking it out on us. Waiting an extra day for the pittance did have quite a knock on effect. Perhaps there would be no bread left and we had very little else in the house to eat.

The milk was delivered daily but paid for every Friday on collection after the round was finished. Fortunately our milkman was a woman and she understood the situation, possibly from a woman's perspective, giving mother an extra day to pay what was due in.

To begin with there was only five shillings sent up for each child, nothing for mother because she was legally allowed to live in his house for free as long as he paid the mortgage. I don't recall this amount ever going up but then again I was only party to the things Mother wanted us to know.

The fact that she never really worked except for some small cleaning jobs meant Mother was never a provider of money into the scenario. It was always said to us kids that if "He" found out she made any money "He" would stop ours coming. I was never sure of the accuracy of her statement but then again she could say anything to us and we had no way of researching the truth.

There was a visit to the solicitors in Manchester one day, not long after Dad left, when I saw him again. Mother and her brood trooped up a flight of dark stairs off Market Street and Alan, Margret and I sat on a landing on those wooden round backed chairs which seemed to be produced in their millions.

All the windows to the offices were frosted glazed and the firm's name was written on them all in stark black letters. I sat looking at them, wondering if it was to stop someone pinching the glass. With their name on it would be difficult to steal the windows, and then put them into your own home now wouldn't it?

The meeting between Mother and dad was to set and seal the legal issues of the separation such as to who was to live where and how much money the children were worth each week.

Later in life I was told the dad would not divorce because in those days it was not constructive when in the nursing profession. It could have hindered his progress up the ladder at the hospital. Besides the divorce court proceedings were gleefully reported in the local press and it was regarded as such a derogatory thing! A legal separation was the best thing to do. How progress has changed society's attitude on such aspects of life and relationships! For better or for worse, is the question? I'm never sure on such things.

Anyway we were always being told that we had no money by mother. This led to a dirge of excuses when things cropped up such as the sound of the ice cream man's 'The Happy Wanderer' to the very occasional activity at school that required finance. New clothes and spasmodic treats were an absolute no go.

Eventually we all got the message and just gave up asking, ignoring any calls the world might give to spend money in it. The cheapest food and household items were always bought and places such as Swinton, Cross Lane or Eccles market were trawled stall by stall for bargains such as the bag of broken biscuits to buy cheap or the least expensive toilet paper.

We even had a lecture on how many sheets to use when going for a 'Number 2'. Incidentally we were told to only take two sheets, fold them together, wipe once then fold them again into themselves and wipe a second time. Strange things to remember for childhood, but I must say

The Weybridge Holiday

I am still not extravagant in many ways, this being one!

The paper we suffered was like grease-proof paper and when I discovered soft tender toilet paper later in life it was a real revelation. "How the other half must have lived?" I thought. With this life style in mind, expensive luxuries such as holidays were just non starters in those days after dad left.

Except for Weybridge! Yes for those who don't know the upper middle class society of this pleasant England, Weybridge is in the Stockbroker belt of Surrey. Now what on God's earth does this dysfunctional, lower working class penniless group of mother and her three children have to connect them with such an idyllic and iconic area of wealth and stability? It was Uncle Gordon.

He was mother's elder and only brother, a good caring man and a God fearing bastion of the local Presbyterian Church. He was unwittingly mother's idolised sibling who was held out to Alan and I as the pinnacle of honesty and truth. "If you could only be more like your Uncle Gordon," was a frequent saying in our house.

To be fair Uncle Gordon was a very good man, good with us kids and he had a great sense of what was right and wrong. He used to do basic magicians tricks that I never knew the answers to.

He lived with his wife and family in a large but tired Victorian semi which he rented and had done since moving to the Vickers Air factory at Brooklands during the war as a fireman.

His long back garden was host to a wonderful old apple

tree and I never got over the fact that I could go and pick windfalls and eat them without paying or having to nick them. Little bright red beauties that the juice ran down the ends of my mouth when I bit into them, so delicious, and free! Yes fruit really did grow on trees in Weybridge, wicked!

Aspects like this made this village a land of milk and honey for us in such austere times. Uncle Gordon was also the fiddler in the family. Not the kind of fiddler I was use to back in Salford but the Scottish fiddle and he would play whilst his sister Annie sang soprano.

This hereditary of skilled Celtic musical talent was a little lost on mother. Saying that, she did not let this lack of skill stop her watching the White Heather Club every Friday night on TV whilst she sang, word perfect to all the Scot's folk and popular songs. Mother would sit with her right foot on the hearth tapping in beat and she would smile, rocking her head in time and singing as if recalling some distant part of her life which was much more pleasant than the one she lived now.

Uncle Gordon was not an affluent man but had a relatively good job in an office somewhere in London. He probably did not waste his money, originating from Aberdeen, but I'm sure he sent the train fare up to Mother so we could travel down to visit him one summer. A treat that had so many offshoots of joy and excitement to this little boy deprived of the riches that travel and seeing the world has to offer. It was another exquisite time when I knew I was not to be beaten, scalded or ridiculed when he, his family or members of the public were within earshot.

The rules had been laid out in Mother's uncompromising fashion. No 'being naughty' at all, 'watch our manners constantly' and we had to 'do whatever she said AT ALL TIMES or we will pay for it when we got back home'.

We travelled on the 57 bus from Swinton Town hall to the centre of Manchester carrying two old battered cases with our clothes in and walked across Piccadilly Gardens to Piccadilly Station. No such trivial bus ride to and Aunts around Manchester this time. We were going on a steam train to London, the big city, the name of a place I knew only in articles described in school books or stories such as Peter Pan read by teachers at school.

Steam trains made such halls of industry as large railway stations exciting sensory places in those days. The gradual crescendo of sensory rush I can recall with such accuracy. Arriving on the station front the sounds bellowed from gaping man-made grotto's to penetrate in front of me.

It was like entering the cavern of a dragon which was steaming and breathing his fire as a warning to all, being dragged into them by Mother.

There are memories of the smell of the engine oil and grease installed in a brain held treasure chest that opens up whenever I visit old steam railways, beaming golden lights of excitement lighting up as the lid of the chest opens up. There is a very special smell that is the mixture of steam and the coal burning in the open furnace that supply's the energy from the very innards of the beast.

Rushing people and whistles sounded by the staff along

with station announcements, it was all a new world, so big and bustling, a cacophony of sound and sensory rush. Sounds of steam ejecting from worn pistons and screaming out of accurately machined whistles were music to my ears.

I had poured my eyes over every page of the pictures in books of trains shunting out of such palaces, or steaming through the darkness of the small hours. Delivering the night mail had come to life in one glorious day; the pictures did not do justice to the real multisensory exhibition I was to revel in.

The rarity of my long distance travel almost made this trip the pinnacle of my life's excitement for me, especially in such a gigantic dirty glass and steel cathedral of sensory stimulation, Piccadilly Station. Honestly, to a small boy such as me it was really every Christmas and birthday wish all rolled into one, right in front of my eyes. To a deprived freckled faced ginger haired kid, with the daily attrition I knew as life, I really was in heaven!

Boarding the train we sat in a carriage that was second class. Second class to me was rich, not like the old third class compartment I had previously travelled on to Southport one summer afternoon from Swinton station.

That was a single carriage with no way out except the two doors at either side. That was a cheap, half day, after lunch ride, that meant we had a tea of Mother's cheese and tomato sandwiches on the beach. Cheese and Tomato sandwiches that always remind me now of the sand that would give the butties a certain 'grit!'

The London train had a corridor and we could walk

about whilst it rushed us across the English countryside to our haven of tranquillity, Uncle Gordon's. It whistled us across the English country side, gaining speed and making its rhythmical clacking sound whilst the wheels sped over the rails. We rocked to its suspension as we tore round smoothly banked corners, past woods, fields and midland towns.

I can even remember getting grit from the engine in my eye when walking past an open window. The smell from the steam that enveloped the grit and came through the open space whilst we were travelling was scrumptious. Well worth a few minutes pain to breath in the light, moist fumes.

On arrival at Euston we were greeted by our silver haired benefactor, Uncle Gordon. He kissed mother on the cheek and gave each of us a warm handshake. Real gentlemen did that sort of thing. Scenes of spontaneous expressions of warm emotions were not something I saw as a child. Whether it was a family trait or a cultural element of the time I'm not sure, I just know it did not happen.

Don't ask me about the weather we encountered or other aspects of the journey across the noisy city that day. I was just glued to the bus window watching the cars, lorries, buses and what looked like millions upon millions of people busily swarming along the streets and pavements, like ants in a newly disturbed nest.

After what seemed like half a lifetime we finally reached our destination at the other terminal station that housed the final journey to our summer utopia. Uncle Gordon ran this final leg as a daily grind to work and back. Today he was in leisure mode and the journey was different for him, shepherding his younger sibling and her children to his abode.

How did you know men in the nineteen fifties and early sixties were on holiday? Easy, no tie around the neck, just the shirt collar placed over the lapels of their jackets. Such a statement made with a straightforward change of everyday wear. How simplistic life was then.

The short walk from Weybridge station to Uncle Gordon's house was one through a strange world of tree lined avenues, a village green and of course the cars that were so instantly different to the ones that trundled around Swinton every day.

Every third mode of transport here seemed to be a rover, jaguar or even a Rolls Royce. These were visual extensions of the value in a person's bank account especially when used to carry out the mundane tasks of collecting a loaf of bread or cakes for tea from the village shops. Many other striking differences to Salford began to reveal themselves such as the bicycles the women used with wicker baskets on the front, used for peddling around the leafy lanes.

The quiet of village life of Weybridge also differed so from the dirty bustling environment I was used to. To me people also spoke with a funny accent and called every one "Dack." 'Caps' weren't placed on your head but filled with tea and drunk from. It seemed such a strange way to talk to this uneducated, untraveled naive northerner, a different language and definitely a different life style.

I probably stuck out like a sore thumb to the locals but was too young and innocent to realise it. Yet this alien to me way of life seemed so natural in this oasis of calm, this bastion of middle England. "How strange." I remember thinking.

The home of my cousins was a tall brick built, hundred year old three story labyrinth of thirties furniture and smelt of beeswax polish. The house was filled with large rooms, big windows and tall ceilings, it really was another world. The front door was located on the side of the house, leaving the front room to be the full width of the building. I never got used to that!

The front door was original, made from solid wood. The top half was enchanting, filled with large coloured glass panes with blue and green mathematical shapes that reflected on the narrow hall carpet when the sun shone on them. The door bell was a worn brass pull knob set into a hollow in the stone frame supporting the entrance.

To the left of the hall was the large front room or parlour that was sparsely furnished with a large red pattern carpet the covered the centre of the highly polished floorboards. This room was little used except for relaxing or reading, two skills I have never managed to master, so I was a very infrequent visitor in there.

The door on the right of the hall way opened up into the back room, where most of everyday life was lived by the family. The radio was in there, next to Uncle Gordon's chair, the clothes rack was suspended from the ceiling over the fire for drying the family's garments and the table was placed against the wall where all the family sat to eat.

This was the very table that educated my taste buds to Chocolate spread for the very first time, such bliss! I still have an inner smile today whenever I treat myself to its seductive charms, spread thickly on wholemeal doorsteps.

Aunty and Uncle would always have their ash tray in the centre of this table almost in constant use. You have to remember in those days smoking did not have the social stigma it has today. The general population was uneducated to its ills. It was before all the research on tobacco's chemical content and carcinogenic properties came out. During the war dad said he even got fifty cigs as part of his wages in the Army, so smoking was ingrained into all of society, even the educated lower middle classes such as Uncle Gordon.

Alan and I slept in one of the top two attic rooms on the third floor up steep winding stairs in a tree top like den with a small solid wood door which opened with a dented brass ball handle. Our awe was enhanced when we were told that when the house was built these were the servant's rooms.

My time on this holiday was spent full of pleasant times, safe and care free and I quickly adapted to this lifestyle Such as playing out in the garden with my older cousin; he played cricket, quite a new sport for me, very upper class!

I knew him already from a previous holiday he had spent with us in Rhyll, a lot older than me but a nice chap. The apple tree in the garden also held wonders of free apples and we were also allowed to play in the local village woods.

Imagine my thought when Aunty said it was there where

some of the Robin Hood TV series was filmed. He was a hero of mine watched every Saturday teatime where he took me into a land of righting wrongs and redistributing the wealth and imbalances of the world. Just the person I wanted in my life to correct the ills and wrongdoings handed out to me on a daily basis.

He actually stood in the wooded area I was in; I just could not wait to get back to school to give myself some street credibility with my peers when I relayed this information to them. Actually the real Robin Hood, here where I now played, my hero!

What a holiday, what a look into Pandora's Box of delights, even if I knew it was not to last and reality was just around the corner. So often there in the upper floor bedroom at night gazing out through the roof window I would ask God above my head to change my life and let me stay here in Weybridge, being loved and not battered, forever.

It was in one of those moments that one of my little friends came to me, up there in the loft room at Uncle Gordon's. He stood in the corner called my name softly, asking me to play, and I just talked to him. Standing there in his soft white night gown he said I will be Ok and that I will be loved. I remember crying and as the tears rolled down my cheeks I wanted to know why I can't just be normal and loved. Why did I have to come here to see what should be then go back to what was the harsh reality of my life.

Back in the daytime my cousin played games with me

an older brother would normally have done, without the pressures of the daily survival of the fittest and canniest.

Cricket became a new joy and I was also introduced to the complex nature of high finance: Monopoly. It was a board game that they all played in Weybridge, of course. It meant I could hold one hundred and five hundred pound notes and in numbers like thousands of pounds. Money like I really never would see, not even today, there in my hands!

When I had time on my own I would go upstairs and lay the board out, take the metal car, the boot, dog and other implements and play my own game, not fully understanding the rules but enjoying handling the money and houses.

Such bliss should never have been put into a few short weeks only to be crashed into reality when landing back at Swinton to the dingy little semi where mother played out her cruelty through the madness on Alan and me.

Should I pinch the board and take it back to Swinton with me? Would it help me to break free of mother and her oppression. Why do my cousins have it when they have all and I need the game so badly? Thoughts like these would cloud my head often when I had time on my own. I was not overt to taking the odd item I desired that was not mine, it's just redistribution of wealth I would justify myself with when my inner conscience questioned the act.

At the time I never saw it as stealing, just the only way I had to become equal to the other people around me in my life who seemed to have it all. It was very common for me in those days to keep something I had not bought or someone else actually owned. The subconscious message from Jesus of equality and looking up to Robin Hood and William Tell on TV gave me an illegal excuse for taking things as a child.

Excuses such as 'no moral leadership' 'lack of strong positive parental influences' 'poor, deprived, single parent dysfunctional family' would today be my claim as I am feebly excuse this behaviour. Difficult and embarrassing for me today as an adult trying to explain to you why I used theft as a child to try to claw back some self worth. It's a habit that has died with my childhood but I still need to come to terms with myself when, at times like this, I have a resurgence of guilt and have to describe, as a mature person, my misdemeanours in a previous life.

One element of the holiday that was to have a profound and lifelong positive effect upon my existence was meeting Penny. She was the daughter of friends of Uncle Gordon and they came around often in the time we were there on holiday.

Penny and I would play in the garden, inventing games and using our imagination to become other characters, as kids do. She was the sweetest most innocent person I had ever met so far in my life and she was so unlike every other person I had seen on this planet.

She does not present herself on the few faded old black and white photos I still have as memory joggers from the day but with hindsight I can possibly understand why. Mother once took me aside and said when there was no one else around that I was to stop watching Penny in the way I was doing. This rule was endorsed with a very sound shake to my torso.

Penny was in her mid teens I guess and just wanted to play with me such childlike games, some of which I had never even known existed. Her body was slightly plump and she had a round spotty face with oval almost slanting eyes. Penny taught me such skills like how to make Daisy chains and I was so fascinated with her different way of being. I also vividly recall a day we all spent on the Thames nearby with us sat on the grass banking talking and playing.

Penny and I played hide and seek in amongst the trees and bushes in the river bank, she had some paper and crayons and we drew together for what seemed like ages. Penny had a childlike innocence that was on a par with mine yet she was so much older. On adult reflection I guess she was just great fun to be with.

Her dress code was always blouses with cardigans over the top, flared style skirts and white ankle socks. Yet I could not help be fascinated by her mystique and persona. It really was like she was from another planet and I subconsciously felt that it was an honour to be asked into her company.

She even smelt different, not excessively pretty like the other female teens that would be self obsessed with their looks and presentation but Penny was just so plainly different in every way. She was, although I never realised at the time, a Mongol. No, not from that far distant land of yurts and mountains but Penny had a condition known today as Down's Syndrome.

I had no concept of her disability then and her status

was never discussed with me. Like so many other things in that age and society, it was not talked about. Her slower cognitive ability gave her an almost inappropriate ability to communicate with people without any social hang-ups.

She was a blessing to be around. She just got on with life and people as if barriers of age or class were just not there. Through knowing her for that short period of time I swear she gave me an interest and empathy that has held me right up to today to be a lecturer for people with disabilities; such was the power of her being herself.

Penny certainly gave me the aspect of not being scared with those who look or behave differently especially in those days when most of the disabled were handicapped by being locked up in hospital and not seen on the streets. Penny was a person I would never forget and will be thankful for the mind opening experience she gave me.

● ● ●

"Do not forget to show hospitality to strangers,
for by doing that some have entertained
angels without knowing it."

Hebrews 13:2

17

Hospital Visit:Number 1

I must also have been a sickly child at times, not that this extracted any long term sympathy from mother. Twice in my childhood I was subject to long hospital stays. The first was after the visit to Dr Smith and his recommendation for adenoids and tonsils out.

In those days some time after your sixth birthday would nearly always automatically herald this operation. It was as if, written in stone somewhere in the National Health vaults. 'All children at the age of six will have their tonsils out – no matter what'. The Matron/Nanny state worked in those days and with the recommendation from Dr Smith, off I trooped on the bus with mother, admittance letter in hand, to Hope Hospital for my intended short stay.

The number 6 route from Partington Lane was run efficiently by the Salford City Transport. It was always large dark green PP3 style bus. Half the front was the drivers cab separate from the rest of the bus, no doors at the back, just an open platform for the conductor to stand and ring the magic bell from under the stairs.

I could never work out how he could ring it, because I did not know there was a bell there. His arm behind his back and finger touching the button for the bell tucked under the stairs. He could control the driver with a simple press of his finger. I just heard that familiar sound which heralded a request for a stop or when rung twice, all clear to set off again.

On arrival at Hope Hospital I was treated to a false start to my stay and, with hindsight, I should have read the signs and not appeared for the second, near fatal visit. We waited in the ward reception area for quite a while then the nurse came to take my temperature before admitting me. This was standard routine.

I had been sat for what seemed like ages very bored with nothing to do, not wanting to move in case Mother chastised me. You know the stance, looking at my shoes, thinking of other things, trying not to smell the smells that put one off hospitals. The heating was on, as expected, but I had not removed my coat whilst waiting, just removed my balaclava and stuck it into my pocket.

Of course when the thermometer was removed from my mouth I was running a slight temperature. My body temperature was too high for me to stay and I was told to go home and return a week later. Boy did I get it going home.

"Why can't you do anything right?" she nagged as we stood at the bus stop. "I will have to arrange for Alan and Margaret to be looked after again next week," she bemoaned, holding my hand as tight as she could to exert pain without having to hit me in such a public place. I was the reason for her anger and she let me now it.

The time for the second visit promptly arrived seven days later and we clambered aboard the Salford City Transport big green number 6 double decker again. I had my pyjamas in a bag and a comic to read, well follow the story lines through the pictures anyway.

What joy to be going away from her for at least a week! No school and no nagging, it was to be fun. How wrong was I in my thoughts of bliss? I should have realised that Chris Stewart never does anything easily nor do things work naturally for his own benefit.

We arrived and I was promptly admitted. Mother was not to stay long, it was Sunday and I was to have the operation the next morning. Visiting times were extremely strict, seven till eight o'clock each evening and no more than three visitors around the bed, with definitely No sitting on the bed.

There was a distinct hangover from Victorian times with rules such as these and they were adhered to with a vigilance and unwavering strictness. The stench of cleanliness and disinfectant always hung around the ward. I suppose I should have been grateful that it masked other smells! Starched uniforms that made nursing staff uncomfortable in their work were also the order of the day. Again it was an establishment that had its own rules that were rigidly adhered to.

Funny how one remembers certain pinpoint moments in the past that caused a rush of fear within one's self. The taste of the pre-op medication left a lasting uncomfortable tinge in my mouth. Going down to theatre was not memorable except from having to wear a night gown that tied at the back!

The gauze being placed over my head and that awful smelling anaesthetic was almost the last I remember of the operation day. Yet how vividly can I recall its placement, then my feeble resistance against at least two of the medical staff as I tried to remove the offending gauze mask. The drops of anaesthetic were applied and I was soon to be unconscious to the world and the work of the surgeon's knife.

Removal of tonsils, adenoids and having my sinus washed out was just another quick job for the operating team but for me it was an attack on my suffering body that my frame did not cope well with at all. I must have been unconscious for a full day, an extended sleep I was not expected to have. Totally unaware of the concerns I had raised in my after operative care I was placed in a bed on the children's ward right under sisters watchful eye.

Being a red head has several visual differences and also some subconscious ones that the mainstream of the population do not have. The temper is one. It's been the bane of my life at the times when it surfaced. I could be playing quite nicely then if a ball shot out from a nearby game and clonked my head I would instantly see red! It's a strange feeling, body and brain taken over by a fight not flight instinct.

One particular day I remember a mock boxing match with another boy in our Drive, Ken. He could afford proper boxing gloves and things such as a full football kit, his dad had his own building business. Ken hit me with a good right hand to my nose, and I went wild. Ken was taller and slightly older than me stronger and always won at play fighting.

This day the red mist came down over my consciousness and I went hell for leather, hitting him with a power I had that came from deep within. He fell over from the strength of my blows and was instantly shocked to realise the worm had turned. It was the temper thing that won the day but I managed to keep it controlled with mother until one night late in my teens but then that's for another day.

Possibly being ginger also meant I had an inadequate ability to heal and congeal when cut which must be another trait. Apparently after the operation in hospital I would not stop bleeding from the area that the offending parts were removed from. I was the cause of great concern initially and was the reason of many visits from the medical staff to my bedside to check up on my progress.

Many years later I was to learn in a conversation with my Moston cousin Sarah how my difficulties were transmitted to other members of the family. She said all the cousins were told that whenever I appeared for the regular day's visit they were never to hit me or let me cut myself because I could not stop bleeding. I was blissfully unaware of this family ruling. What fun I could have instigated for myself if I had known then!

Back on the ward I was watched constantly and a nurse was assigned to visit me at least every half an hour. I drifted between sleep and semi consciousness for what seemed like an age loosing blood at a concerning rate. With reflection I was glad not to be at home, the constant changing of blood stained sheets and pillows would not have endeared me to mother, irrespective of my poor physical well being.

The main outward sign to the rest of the world about how ill I actually was is the relinquishing of an unbending rule. I was placed on the 'free visiting' list. This was a title given to patients who were so ill they could be visited at any time from ten in the morning. This was reserved for very special cases. I must have been very ill although blissfully unaware of my predicament. I stayed on the ward for about six weeks until I was allowed to return home in a somewhat weakened and feeble state.

There were two main perks of staying in hospital for so long. The obvious one was being away from mother and her ranting. The second was seeing my dad. He had left under the cloud of working nights at Hope Hospital, the very place where I was having my care. Well, every night he was on shift I would get to see him, what a bonus. His role was in charge of the nursing staff and he would have his rounds through the night of checking on everyone's wellbeing. This obviously included the children's ward and he would call over to see me. We did not talk much, as if he was keeping his professional role separate from his private one. It was enough for me to get that warm feeling that I had seen and talked to him without the after effect of mother knowing and the consequences of her anger.

I was not to see or contact him again for many years until just before he died. After this hospital visit he was just to remain the target of mother's verbal abuse thrown at us on regular occasions for many years. She did quiz me on my return home about if I had seen him. I just denied his presence saying I was asleep every night. Lies can sometime stave off far greater troubles. Something I learnt at an earlier age but only if I could get away with them!

18

Punishment in the Winter Elements

Another particular memorable night was the night of the cold snow and the underpants. During the 1950's and early 60's we knew the house in Stonegate Drive was an ice box inside so outside would be even colder. Westerly winds prevailed from across the Lancashire plane and their cold streams seemed to hit our house head on. They rushed through the gap between the two houses that stood at the bottom of our small garden making it even colder. In winter, snow lasted sometimes for several weeks, long after it had turned grey from the incessant and innocuous belching of muck from the factories of Trafford Park.

One winter I remember it snowed and stayed frozen for months and months. Most winters from the inside of our unheated bedroom Alan and I could inscribe our initials with our fingernails on the ice that had formed inside the badly fitting metal framed windows. Yet this exposure to the elements was not enough to steel Alan and I against the night we were nearly frozen by having to stand as punishment in the bitter cold.

The precise details for the misdemeanour are unclear in my memory. It could have been reading with the light on, a sibling tiff or just a book falling from the bed onto the floor after 'lights out'. Irrelevant now but the consequences then were sufficient to cause a carving into the subconscious that has remained forever trapped in my memory. A memory that resurfaces whenever I feel the bitter cold or watch stories of Arctic explorers trapped on the ice on the TV.

Mother often quietly stalked up the stairs when she was trying to catch us out. She did it in such a way we never heard her coming. This particular night she crept with her usual stealth then pushed opened the bedroom door to reveal her slim silhouette against the landing light. This outline always terrified Alan and I and we knew that one or other of us was in for it or we were going to get nagged at for however long mother decided she needed to correct us.

She started and this particular night we were not to lay there listening to her constant vilification and character assassination of us. She meant action!

We normally slept in pyjamas and in winter had a jumper on as extra insulation. In the coldest periods we put Dad's old army coat on top of the bed. We still felt cold and it took the mental power of Colossus some mornings to slip out of that bed warmed by our bodies and enter the freezer we called the bathroom.

This night we were dragged out of bed and slapped across the room. Then she demanded we stripped off our clothing and threw us downstairs in just our underpants. She was going to teach us a lesson we were never to forget. She was going to beat the devil out of me, as she pushed me towards the cold outside. Freezing as we were it was nothing in comparison to the temperature drop we were to encounter.

"Outside," she screamed in fury. "Outside you little bastards." We were bundled, pushed and smacked out of the back door and into the cold snow on that dark winter night.

Now the reason for this regular unleashing of anger and torrent of blows was not clear then, and is only partly understood by me today. I think, after years of reflection in idle moments when I have felt strong enough mentally to relive my painful history, that her motivation was either one of two evils. Punishment leads to correction or venting my anger on them will make me feel better and it may also make them behave in the process. The third reason, an illness within her head was not contemplated then but with further reflection possibly the real reason.

How a once quiet, kind and intelligent child who progressed to nursing sick and dying people could turn into this evil centrifuge of power and control I never will, and never want to, understand.

Outside Alan and I went, both crying, and mumbling how

sorry we were. We were marched down the short path on the snow into the back garden.

"Now stay there until you have learn some sense," with a final torrent of blows on both of us she went back into the relative warmth of the house to sit by the back room window watching her two children slowly start to feel the effects of the bitter winters night. How long we there I cannot recall. I do remember Alan cursing and telling me to keep jumping up and down to keep warm. Unfortunately because mother had seen him talking to me she came back again to lash out and stop us from communicating to each other.

Cold, do you know what that word really means? Maybe you are one of the unfortunates who have been trapped in below zero temperatures for whatever reason. I hope, with all I believe in, that you were not suffering the edges of hyperthermia as a punishment inflicted by some overpowering maniac hell bent on total control and the suppression of innocent childhood explorations.

I grew colder and colder, my little body not capable of protecting itself especially with no clothing on except my underpants to protect my dignity. Dignity? What was that in this my existence of cruelty, shame and pain? Stood there in just my underpants outside, what was dignity?

The skin covering my bones was alive with goose pimples. My thoughts ran amok around my increasingly chilly head as my tears froze to my cheeks. Was I ever going to go to school again? Would she ever let me back in? Was I going to die and more importantly when was she going to die?

These thoughts I recall because my mind was galvanised by hatred and survival. Later in my professional learning as a nurse Maslow's Hierarchy of Needs fascinated me and I often relived that night of snow and underpants trying to dissect and find reason in her actions. How my needs that night were just for physical survival and safety, the lowest and most basic form of need according to Maslow.

"Suffer the little children to come unto me," Jesus taught. I often wondered at this phase. Why was the word suffer in there? Knowing the words meaning as I did, How did He really mean it?

My feet and hands were blue and numb, I snivelled and shivered consistently, cried quietly and the salt of my tears felt almost warm against my lips. I blotted Alan out of my mind concentrating only on selfish thoughts of survival.

Whether Margaret was watching or not I cannot recall but later in life she told me she did and she felt such strong emotions of sorrow and suffering for us. She remembers watching in fear from the upstairs window in my bedroom. She was scared in case she was caught by mother and sent to suffer the same fate. Such fear has lasted her lifetime tucked away in her memory.

From Mother's perspective what reason or outcome was required on that night I never knew. Was an apology needed? Should I go to the window and plead on my knees? Was I really sorry or did I just want relief from this grief? Even today I cannot look at her actions then understand her motives.

Punishment in the Winter Elements

I wonder if aspects of incidents like this one steeled me for life's blows that I would encounter later. This physical and mental endurance at such an early age could be recalled later in times of stress with a 'Well I've had worse and survived' as the flip answer to a difficulty. Or did it give me a weakness that makes me stressed? What did she get out of it and why did she do it were questions I never reflected on for long.

Trying to understand her mind was impossible when at the time concentration on survival was paramount. Maybe you have answers. I don't and frankly I do not look for or need them. I only need the conviction to use these extreme incidents to make counterbalances ensuring the world is filed with love and fairness today. I must offer both these positive elements wherever I go, in whatever I do. I cannot bear any injustices nowadays, often I cry softly when I see children dying of famine on the television.

In my professional life I feel I now fight for the rights and well being of people with profound disabilities with an energy that comes maybe from the injustices doled out to me. The nights I watched the peace marches in the southern USA when the black population only wanted a just and fair society. To be able to sit in peace on a public bus was an unjust desire? I had so much empathy for their cause and understood their pain and emotions.

Learning about the slave trade and the people crossing the Atlantic in the holds of those horrendous slave ships I had an emotional reaction driven through my own experiences. Understanding about the Jews, Gypsy's and other persecuted people in Hitler's concentration camps also had a very personal element for me as I discovered about their plight. My realisation that those with learning disabilities were one of the first blocks of people to suffer elimination by Hitler also caused me great grief. My own torture was short lived in experience but long lived in my reaction to others who suffered at the hands of evil, bullying or injustice.

The world, as I see it, has two main problems. It does not share its food fairly and man does not look man in the eyes and each see each other as a brother or equal willing to share their skills, knowledge, resources and love for each other.

Remembering that night in the snow and cold about how we got back into the house is impossible. I just recall the punishment. How long we were there or how it all ended I cannot recollect. I just know I survived and the memory of the pain is easily recalled. How sad when it is only moments or hours like these that you can recall about your mother.

If you are a parent, remember to dot your child's memory with activities of pleasure and love so that in their later life they will recall you with fondness and return love that is real and true.

● ● ●

"No-one has the right to make me feel inferior
unless I consent."

(Eleanor Roosevelt/Princess Diaries I)

19

Whit Walks and Summer Days

Seasonally I much preferred the summer and warmer months, which brought extended freedom and days playing out in the woods or open fields. Whit week heralded the beginning of what I knew as summer.

Whit, a holiday just after Easter, was the only time you got new clothes as kids. The clothes were for the Whit Walks. Every town in the Manchester area had its Whit Walks where the churches turned out to parade with their different organisations around the boundaries of their parish, showing their Christian faith to all.

Swinton which is my part of Salford in west Manchester was no exception. The whole town would turn out to see the bands and marchers go by. I was a member of the church choir but also in the Church Lads Brigade (CLB). Those facts meant I had choices every Whit in Swinton as to which part of the church parade I would be in.

Being in the CLB also meant I learnt to play a drum and was a part of the band. I gained much self credibility at a tender age and it also paid dividends financially. As I marched around, proud as punch, banging out rhythms to the bugler's tunes, neighbours and family friends would line the streets to watch. It was free entertainment really but if they saw you they would run out and drop a three penny bit or sixpence into your new jacket or your pristine uniform pocket. I could make a tidy little fortune, "Just showing off and banging a bloody drum," as mother used to call it. Still I loved it.

I continue to have an affinity to military and brass bands that lasts today and still love tapping rhythms out with my fingers on stretched skin. It makes those tiny little hairs on the back of my neck stand to attention when I hear native drumming or a polished brass band strike up. The full treatment given to some of the classics by a good brass band cannot be beaten into second place by any other form of music. Bands are steeped into my personal history.

What would I have done if I'd have lived down south? "No tradition that lot," I often thought. "Southerners never knew how to have a good time." Southern England was a desert with no Whit Walks, no brass bands and no chips, steak puddings and mushy peas.

Alan and I were also trebly lucky being in the CLB and the fact that our nearest cousins lived in Moston, north Manchester. That meant that Whit Sunday we marched in Swinton with our own church and on Trinity Sunday we could go up to Moston and march with them and their church. Alan and I also used to back up a Church Lads Brigade in Salford at St Clements, join their band and march around Manchester City Centre on Whit Monday. Wow! Did we have a ball of a time, parades, bands, pomp and majesty!

It cost us time spent cleaning our uniforms and my drum would need almost half a tin of Brasso so I could see my face in it before each parade. Shoes were also polished to military precision and the creases in the pants of our uniform were razor sharp. This flurry of cleanliness, spit and polish with military like parades always heralded the start of my summer.

At my tender age in the nineteen fifties there were other ways you knew when summer had come. My bedroom and in fact whole the house was devoid of a cold chill in each room and the frost was gone from inside the windows. The fire was never lit and cousins would come from their respective corners of Manchester for a visit. They would play out with you all day whilst mother and her sister nattered and caught up on the family gossip.

Your clothing would also change. Mother would automatically decide on a particular day of her choosing that summer had arrived. It would always be sometime in the Whit holidays. She would put away my dark grey and heavy short winter pants, the poorly knitted and very naff jumpers and out would come a cotton tee shirt, short grey socks, black pumps and those infamous khaki shorts.

I suppose we wore khaki shorts because they were hard wearing and practical. Unfortunately my sparrow thin legs moved around in them as I played out whilst the light brown material never flinched. Each leg had as much room to move around in as the striker inside the church bell! The other thing was they were such a light colour that if you happened to dribble after visiting the toilet then everyone knew for half an hour after, except you! The only compensation I had was that everybody wore them, and I mean everybody.

In those days designer clothes had not been invented for the masses. Prosperity after the war years had not yet trickled down to the ordinary working classes. If ever you saw a label on someone's clothing then you knew they had their clothing on inside out!

I could also play out all day in the summer time in those halcyon days. Manchester in the late fifties and early sixties was a relatively safe place for me out of doors and parents only warned their children about the road and against getting lost during the long school holidays.

It was a fact that parents would give the defining line: "Be home before the street lights come on." It is said that the children brought up in the Fifties were the last to have a real 'childhood of innocence'.

These untroubled days for the children were to be ended for me because of a notorious Manchester couple, Ian Brady and Myra Hindley, the Moors Murderers. In the mid nineteen sixties young children suddenly started to go missing, plucked off the streets of greater Manchester, never to be seen again. As the horrendous crimes accumulated there was a direct effect on the streets. Children began to stop playing out and roaming the streets and parks of Greater Manchester.

A fear had crept over them instilled by caring and protective parents. Youngsters were beginning to feel unsafe and were either watched continually playing in their own streets or not allowed out at all. Summer holidays became quieter in the streets of Manchester. A fear had begun to cover them and those playing out in them.

Fortunately for me I was old enough not to be concerned at the time the murderous duo were hatching their evil plots. A few years earlier I could and would play out from just after breakfast till suppertime. A few slices of bread wrapped in the grease proof wrapper and an old screw top Dandelion and Burdock pop bottle filed with water were my substance for the day. I did not care, I was off on my bike, hunting wildlife in Wardley or Worsley woods or playing in the streams of the Clough.

My life seemed to be idyllic until I came home too late and was in line for the usual punishment for being in past seven at night. Having a watch of your own in those days was absolutely unthinkable. I had to rely on asking strangers or being in a position where I could see the large town hall clock from Swinton Town Centre. I soaked up the punishment of being hit and stood for a few hours whilst I was 'nagged'. It was little enough when all I knew I could return the next day to enjoy another full summer day of adventure, fantasy and life in the open.

20

Winter and Those 'Thank You' Letters

I disliked winter for the cold and its enforced encampment with mother in the house. You may be thinking that winter brings the joys of Christmas with peace and good will to all men. Christmas for me had hidden meanings and activities to further expose my curse and extend mother's bag of corrective tricks.

Christmas morning was often OK, presents and mother getting up late, but with the unspoken dread of what was to come, those blasted 'Thank you' notes. Each Aunt and Uncle mostly sent us postal orders for about half a crown. I would love trotting down to the sub post office at the bottom of Partington Lane to exchange them for little plastic toy soldiers or metal cars.

I once owned a small die cast Bentley Continental with suspension and doors and a boot that opened! It was richness in miniature to me and often I would sleep with it tucked under my pillow after having taken it around the Mediterranean coast on the lino in my bedroom. That car did some miles over the worn flooring but many more in my head. Anyway back to Christmases.

On Boxing day out would come a Basildon Bond writing pad, pencils for me, best biro pen for Alan and Mother would make us write thank you notes to her family that had been so kind as to send money or a present. This was fine for the other two, Alan and Margaret but well can you imagine the spin it put me into?

Normally one of the old high back wooden dining chairs with brown plastic seats was turned to face me, a mat or large book placed on the seat to rest the paper on as a make shift desk. I was then expected to write very neatly to this kind Aunt or Uncle telling them how I enjoyed their present or what I wanted to spend the money on.

On my knees leaning the paper against a book I would try to get the letters right and spell correctly. Always under very close scrutiny. Mother would start off by pointing out to me the spellings and unreadable writing.

The only way I could write a word I did not know was for her to say each individual letter out loud, wait for me to write it then deliver the next. This was painfully slow and it did not have the desired effect for correct spelling. Letters, especially vowels, were always in the wrong place, some were not supposed to be there and others from the land of Mars landed into the words. Patience was not one of mother's virtues! She would soon tire and start to remonstrate with me about how lazy I was and how easy it should be for me to learn.

"Why can't you do it, the others can? You're just lazy and don't listen," she would scream at me. Time and time again I worked so hard to get the letters the right way around, let alone stress about the neatness of the writing under the close scrutiny of Mother. When this system failed because of my inabilities the page was ripped out of the pad, screwed up, thrown on to the fire then I was shouted at to try again.

The element of wasting paper when we were so short of money was another issue brought into the argument. It never took long before the nagging and insults turned into physical correction of the smacking kind. Sometimes it would be when I had contradicted her or tried to justify my wrongdoings. Whack! I felt her hand across my head. How I hated those pencils and posh paper. That light blue pad I can still visualise today and when I see an old dinning chair turned away from the table like an impromptu desk well, the ghost of my Christmas past is always ready to haunt me.

One time in particular I was really struggling. Even today, I still have good and bad days with my dyslexia. The curse can affect me in waves, some times the tide is strong, sometimes it recedes. Writing this page today I will soon know if I cannot string anything together well and have to just leave the story.

The F7 button on the laptop gets very warm on days like this. Added to this is my total inability to plan logically which further compounds my problems.

You may feel reading this book that some things are somewhat out of sequence. You could be right, I cannot place a clear and organised chronological order into my daily doings or planning. I have had to read and re read these words you are reading so often to try to get a more organised flow. Apply this to writing a letter, especially when much younger, and 'whoosh' things are placed in such a random order and got scribbled down as they enter my head. Random thoughts lead to random writings!

I now go and potter in the greenhouse or get out into the outdoors for a walk or some practical task if I can. Nothing will correct this scrambling or surge of inability to write legibly by hand, until it goes away on its own.

Ask my line manager about the days when I seem to just put a tiny millipedes foot worth in my work and produce havoc in my wake! I create disasters in virtually every other thing I say and do. I break this and drop that, miss key words that are said to me or forget something extremely important. All innocently and unknowingly done of course until I am pulled up about it! Don't ask me why, I will never know exactly what goes wrong in my head but that is just the way the curse affects me today. Good days mean I can get through the day without any great catastrophe. Bad days can be disastrous.

This particular day trying to write to benevolent family was a painful disaster. If only I had the knowledge of myself that I have today and the power to explain adult to adult with her who controlled my life so violently.

21

Contact with Dad and His Side of the Family

Mother initially had not been in a good mood. Early on after dad had left he would, through his sister Patty, ask us what presents we wanted. I occasionally saw my Aunt Patty when she visited Dad's family around the corner from us at the bottom of Partington lane.

I will now have to explain some of the complexities of Dad's family. His mother had numerous children. I now know because I have drawn up the family tree. For reasons best known to her and left in the past her sisters brought up some of the later ones. A common task in the days of extended families that all lived in close proximity to each other, especially in the small terraced streets of Salford.

Now the lady I knew as Jen was explained as Dad's cousin. She married a Swinton man, James, who ran his family engineering business. Jen and James lived in what was James' Dad's house, a large detached thirties built house. James was wealthy enough to have a boat moored somewhere in Wales, a caravan which the family had numerous holidays in and the family engineering firm.

Their house had an extension and a wooden floor which went from the back of the house through to the front room. Far more importantly to me James was the owner of a loft which had a complete model train set in. He once treated me to a visit and I stood in awe as his trains ran all around the room on three tracks, through miniature stations and fields of minute plastic sheep. It was a little boys dream.

We were called to visit them at times such as when their two delightful little girls were born, the only cousins I knew on my Dad's side, Shelia then Tracey. Jen was the only sort of regular contact with Dad's side and it was explained somewhat sketchily that she was Dad's cousin.

"So what does that make Shelia and Tracey to me?" Whenever I asked the answers from mother were vague. They are actually my cousins but for reasons to be explained later never revealed as such in those days.

In essence Olga brought Jen up and was called Mam by Jen. When the time came for Jen to apply for a passport it conspired that Dad's mother was also mother to Jen making her Dad's sister, not cousin! She had passed her over to Olga just after birth for Olga to bring Jen up as her own, the child being blissfully aware of her parentage.

Jen's real name on her birth certificate was actually Ivy, and she was really my Dad's half sister. Half because my grandmother had three different partners in her life time and produced possibly eleven or twelve children! Confused? Can you imagine how I felt trying to unravel the complexities of Salford life in the early 1900's with how my mind works! It did simplify my relationship with Shelia and Tracey, cousins with whom I am still in regular contact with today.

One particular fateful year I asked through Patty for Dad to get me a set of army trucks for Christmas. Mother was fuming. When I told her what I wanted she really let rip. I really wanted some toy die cast army vehicles.

"Bloody army, I hate the army," she yelled and let me know in her usual way how I should correct my views. The nagging about killing people with guns and how the Army were both evil were fired at me on many occasions.

Still, somehow that Christmas day I received several boxed, model army metal trucks, tanks and land rovers. Eagerly I opened the boxes. This was far more presents than I had previously received, each new box revealed a new delight to me that filled my little heart with joy and pride. All were brand new and pride of place was given to the ambulance with the great Red Cross on each side against its regulation green. It also had two doors at the back that swung open. It was a dream.

All that Christmas day I played and played with the trucks, they filled my time and left no thoughts for the cold in the room where I transferred my play through my mind to far flung places with them. Under the chairs and cushions I had the army convoy moving though India and

Burma along the carpet, then across the lino floor towards Japan. What I was really doing was replicating the places I'd heard my dad had gone to in the last war. I had mixed a cake of destruction from a real life recipe of disaster.

Mother must have watched and fumed, her anger building up as I innocently played. "Why do you want to copy Jim? I'll show him. The bastard, thinks he can lord it over the kids, influencing them from his place in Weaste," she must have thought. Tired from the land battles I had played out all day I parked up the convoy under a chair in the front room as their make shift barracks.

The next day, Boxing Day I ran downstairs, quickly ate my cereal then flew into the front room to continue winning World War 2. I looked for my convoy of brand new toys. They were not parked in the barracks where I had left them. I started to search around under the furniture and went into the back room.

The back room, where most of this day was to be acted out, was a dingy place. It had a worn carpet square that covered the centre of the floor. Between the edges of the carpet and the wall was the brown lino that got a regular clean and polish making it a great slide when I only had my socks on, and Mother was not around.

The furniture was plain and slightly tatty and the wallpaper was of faded squares with light coloured flowers on. A heavy square of dark brown wallpaper was next to the door where it protected the wall from those like me who rubbed the wall as we entered. An old wooden fold up table was always placed on the wall opposite the fireplace and chairs were dotted into convenient spaces, filling the area with a pale, brown tiredness.

The fire was the single aspect of warmth and was only lit in very cold weather. The room had a feel of a depressive lack of money. This was one of the three main rooms that played stage to many of my corrective sessions with Mother. Maybe, just maybe, Mother had seen the goodwill of Christmas and tidied my new toys away for me.

Sadly that was not the case. Mother was sat near the fire with her foot tapping on the hearth. A bad sign! "If you are looking for your bloody army things I've thrown them in the bin," was her remark as I entered. "I bloody well told you all day yesterday if you leave them out I will bin them, you little bastard."

Several times in my life as a child I was rocked to the core by mother and this time was one of them. It was like falling into a pit, totally dark, no sides to grab to steady the fall and with a destination at the end that heralded the fires of Hades.

In that fall I was filled with a fear and panic that sent my senses absolutely haywire and my stomach sickly. I had no control over these feelings or their consequences. This time no hits, slaps or punches, no thrashing with her belt, initially just words and one action. Did I hear her right?

"But mum I put them all away last night. I parked them up under the chair," I cried in disbelief.

"That's right you left them out on the lino for anybody to trip up over them. I bloody well told you that I would do it and I keep my word." I sank to my knees, she showed a mean streak that cut me continually to the bone. The only time I ever had an army set of cars and trucks and 'SHE' has put them in the bin, wiped them from the face of this earth because 'HE' sent them. I was an unwitting, powerless pawn in a power game between two adults, one of which ran a continuous campaign of hatred and bitterness against the other.

This day was to be a gigantic disaster in the tragic life of Christopher Stewart and to be remembered and recalled for many years after. How could she do this? I loved those little trucks with a passion? Was it because I loved them, because they are army or because my dad sent them? With the hindsight of age and experience I would bet she was livid that my father sent me army trucks.

How she hated the army, it was part of the cause, in her mind, part of the breakup of her marriage. How she hated Jim, her husband, who left her with three kids to bring up, the boys difficult to say the least. How she must have hated me, the bad penny in her change and cause of so many rants and rages because I was naughty, nay more than that, evil. How she must have loved tipping those small metal toys symbols of so much she hated, into the bin. Satisfying in that it hurt the two people she despised the most.

That action must have been sweet revenge for her. Little I was to say, just a cry of remonstration about how could she destroy the Christmas presents sent via his sisters. Mother now had the bit between her teeth and she was not going to let me go. In her mind I need to right the wrong of loving those army trucks.

She made me get the chair out from the dining set and turn it around. Now I was to write to her sisters and brother to thank them for the 'real' presents I had received, from her side of the family. The pad and pencils appeared. "Now get bloody writing!" she exclaimed. "I want you to tell Uncle Gordon and Aunty Alice how much you liked their postal orders and not a word about those bloody army trucks."

I know I felt many feelings that moment. I was angry, helpless, bitter, defeated and most of all evil for loving something which in Mother's eyes, was so wrong. My mind was also stressed to the extent that dyslexia would have overridden any thoughts and actions of normality and order.

I know today so well how stress affects the thought patterns in my brain, I can't read or write half as well and all rational thoughts of order can go right out of my mind. Dyslexia kicks in like a bullet going through tissue paper as I feel the stress levels rise. Today I can control this affect by walking away from paperwork or computer based issues, then, as a child I was trapped by one much more powerful than I, mother.

She leant over me as I tried to place the right words on the paper. I was shaking and my mind was all over the place. Would those letters form correctly? Would they heck! I tried to get lines moving to resemble the letters I needed for her words and even place the letters in the correct order. The stress in my heart rapidly affected my mental state and with that the trigger that enhanced my dyslexic traits. Tears dripped from my cheeks to spoil the ink and make an even greater justification for mother's annoyance.

Letter after letter I wrote was unacceptable. The more I tried the more it went wrong and the more pressure she piled on me. Her hand must have hurt with all the times it was stopped in full flight against the side of my head. I was in a free fall, careering into the blackest pit I had been in for such a long time.

The joys of Christmas, peace and goodwill to all, were lost on me that day and for a long time after. Finally as she reached top pitch and I was told that I was the reason for her to feel this way as she dragged me away from the chair. "I will beat this devil out of you. You little bastard! Christopher Stewart you are evil enough to make a saint swear," she screamed.

By this time my knees hurt from the pressure of kneeling there. One of her most sadistic moments was about to begin when my hair was used to lever me up to attention. "I'll make you write properly with that pencil you lazy little bastard," her face was so close to mine, I felt her every breath and spit as she screamed her insults at me.

She let go her grip and went to the sideboard, top right draw; I knew it so well as the holder of the belt. I knew I was to get leathered with the belt again, I just knew it. Today she was angry enough to use the buckle end. My body tensed in fright. Then I stopped and through my tears saw her with a hand full of pencils. What was to be my fate?

"I'll teach you," she kept repeating and threw the pencils on the old brown lino floor next to the ill fitting French window. They spread all over the polished surface. She bent down and placed them on their sides in a flat line to cover a small square on the floor in front of the chair. "Now kneel on them," I hesitated and received her hand sharply on my head as a reminder to do as was ordered. "Kneel there, you liar, saying you can't use them, Alan can use them, Margaret can use them, everybody on God's earth can use them, and so can you, you lazy bastard. I'll teach you," each part of her shouting was emphasised with a lash of her hand.

How was I to get out of this predicament? I could not write properly especially today, I had a curse, exasperated by my emotional state. I just wanted to run away and die.

"No, no don't hit me, don't make me do it, please," I pleaded with my tormentor, "I'm so sorry I will never, ever, do it again." This was my feeble attempt to get her to retreat from the emotive state she was in. I remember trying to alter the situation for myself by shouting these things.

Fighting back in such a manner only brought more strength from her and another flush of anger narrowed into more blows at me. I slid and slipped over the shiny lino. She followed my body moves with accurate blows. Grabbing my hair again I was pulled over the untidy pile of leaded wood.

"Now kneel and try to think how you can write properly." I lowered myself quickly onto the pencils and even my slight body weight was sufficient to produce pain in my knees. "There's nothing wrong with you, the others can do it so can you. You are just lying and I hate liars. You can kneel there until you can write those letters properly," she screamed.

The others were Margaret and Alan. At times like this they went to ground, understanding that when mother was on one, most commonly at me, then you stayed away listening to the screaming and sobbing at a distance. It was better not to be within eyeshot or you could be instantly dragged in to the nagging and any wrong doing from recent history would be used as an excuse to help unleash her anger on you.

Mother retired to the couch and sat down. She panted with all her exertions. Then started to cough again, spluttering and bringing up small amounts of phlegm.

"You made me do this, why do you make me feel this way?" I was told. More guilt poured over me but it did not help me to get away from this situation. My knees really started to hurt; I could feel the imprint of the pencils through my skin. The very bones in my legs were pressing against the wooden lead carriers and all the weight of my body was forced into that small area of my knees.

The pain was soon to be incredible for me but I held up for some time until I could not take it any longer. In all this agony I would have done anything for a release, freedom from the torture I endured. Why was I being made to hurt for something I could not control, correct or even understand? My curse again made me pay for my disability. I tried to stand up, crying to Mother that it really hurt me. "Get back down till you have learnt how to use them properly," she yelled as she got up and pushed me back to the pencils again. They rolled as my knees hit them and scattered over the floor. My knees hit the hard lino covered wooden floor with a resounding thump. They were red by now and took over the whole of my thought processes.

Christmas always meant some form of punishment to me. All three of us knew it was a flash point for Mother, sending her over the top somehow. This Christmas my suffering was pushed to its extreme.

The thought of dying and floating up to heaven in blissful warmth with no sounds of screaming or pain occasionally comforted me at these times. Never had I wanted it more than now. I knew I was to endure further because the letters had not yet been written. Could I just not stop people sending me anything for Christmas? Perhaps I could have some brain surgery that would make me read and write properly. It would change all this and end many hours of endurance and suffering to me. I was, after all, really a kind boy who just wanted to live with nature and look after animals, did she not see that?

My special friends never came to me when Mother was in the same room, just comforted me after the event of torture. Perhaps Mother could just die. Could I kill her and get away with it? I would have to run away and live on the moors above Manchester or in the woods down the road.

Any long term solutions to my predicament were quickly

banished when she hit me again and I was immediately brought into line with the crisis I was actually in. "Get to that bloody chair and write properly, I'm fed up with you and your bleeding laziness and excuses," she still snorted her anger, how could such a simple matter of writing a few thank you notes be such a life or death matter?

I knelt again on the floor, this time against the dinning chair and felt the pain shoot back into my legs. I could not see well and my tears were wetting the paper.

She must have exploded and hit me so hard with her hand that I fell over and I crashed to the floor. "I'll beat some sense into you and the devil out of you before I'm done." This was one of her standard phrases at a time like this. I knew I could not do anything she wanted today; I just wanted to curl up and die. It would be such sweet relief. My release came in such an unexpected way. The next order surprised me.

"Get to bed, go on get to your room and stay there until you can act sensibly and can thank people for sending you proper presents. Get those clothes off and get to bed." At the time I did not realise my luck but just took myself off up the flight of stairs and went towards my bedroom snivelling and crying like a wounded cat.

The day had not reached its middle, yet here I was being sent upstairs to spend the rest of Boxing Day away from the others. I was miserably tired and ready to hide from her and the world under my bed sheets.

I just cried and cried, softly and with a self-pity that was so great I just wanted to go to sleep and never wake up. Often I had this feeling. It was usually when I had been given a really good beating and for what something that I knew I could not have changed.

I lay for ages there, under the sheets waiting for her to reappear, as was her want. Often I had been stood in the hall for hours whilst she nagged me with the occasional lashings thrown in. Then she would wait for a short while open the bedroom door with the hall light on and start nagging again. She could go on and on dragging up times when I had done this and that, giving example after example of my wickedness then shouting how ashamed she was of me then what I would be in for if I ever did things such as them ever again.

I would often be kept awake till two in the morning as she went through this repertoire. Yes I was scared of her and feared the lashings especially from her belt but I also hated her. Hated her with a passion, felling trapped in this world of punishment for all my wickedness and humility around what I now know as my disability but then was my laziness and stupidity. This hatred was one of the reasons I had strength enough to help me cope through the worst of times.

She was my mother and I just wanted her to be normal or dead. It was my curse that caused it and I just wanted to be ordinary, just like everyone else. I just wanted a kind mother that I could love and to be able to read and write properly. Was I asking too much? Was this all part of some vast plan that would give me the steely courage to endure life's difficulties I was to encounter? Why me?

"Please just let it all go away," I cried that horrible day. Then the soft voice called me from my teary stupor.

"Chris," it called and I knew I had a small friend under the bed to talk to. To cry to and ask the questions of life or death that ran through my mind. My small friend came to comfort me again in my hour of need. I thanked God for this support. They were in my bedroom waiting for mother to go quiet and then they talked to me.

"Chris," I heard. "It will be alright and go away, don't worry." In pain I leant over the side of the bed and saw that comforting sight of my friend, arms open beckoning me to put my mind into a better place. I slept after a while, my body warmed from my own heat under the sheets and hungry from missing two meals but content that I was not to be hit again that day and my special friend to comfort me.

22

The Secret Smokers

Why mother allowed me to roam free all day every holiday in spring, summer and early autumn was, at the time, never in my thoughts. With the hindsight I have today I can see why she wanted me out of her sight.

Imagine why I, playing out all day long, would be such a blessing for her? It really meant she also could indulge in her hidden pastime confidently so that I would never know her surreptitious habit. You see Mother was a secret smoker, the neighbours, her friends, not even her sisters or brother knew.

Why she kept her addiction hidden I will never know. She did tell the world she lived off very little money and that would ply some sympathy from her circle of people she knew. If they also knew she had money for cigarettes then perhaps they would not be so benevolent in keeping her children clothed and given the occasional treat. Who knows what went on in mother's head?

I sussed she smoked when I was about eight or nine. One day I found a packet of Park Drive fags in her pinny pocket as it hung on the nail behind the pantry door. I put them back realising who's they were, quelling my excitement about finding out her secret. Earlier I had started smoking, well before the legal age, scrounging a drag whenever I could off my brother or his mates.

Suddenly, I realised I could use this packet to elicit free fags for myself. I knew she would never openly ask who had stolen any cigarettes from it because that would bring her secret out into the open. It was a fool proof plan that I thought was my passport to a continual supply of free cigarettes.

But, she knew about it all right. Little did I understand then that mother would only vent her anger at me about this when she caught me out for other misdemeanours.

23

Church

My only other regular reprieve, especially in the winter months, for a few hours as a young child at this traumatic time, was when I went to Church. Not that Jesus was uppermost in my thoughts for solace but He did give me a building to visit as a sanctuary on a regular basis.

I joined St Peter's choir at around six years of age as a boy soprano. This was to prove an earthly and heavenly blessing; not that I could sing but being in the choir gave me a dream place to visit every Sunday.

Far more importantly at that time it financed me when I sang. I would receive the princely sum of half a crown at weddings on most Saturdays. Towards the end of the tax year in March we could sing for up to five weddings on a Saturday, it was a religious gold mine.

Twice each Sunday I would dash off up Partington Lane,

surplice in hand to relish the delights of listening to, or more commonly daydreaming during the sermons of the Cannon. But even in my religious attire I could cause my own special brand of havoc.

I recall going home via the Indoo's, one evening in the dark. The Indoo's was the large wild open area behind the Town Hall. Many years previously the area right in the centre of Swinton had been a children's home but then the buildings knocked down to provide the land for the Civic Centre. It also housed a large concrete underground Air raid shelter built for the war. This and the many trees it held there were another adventure playground for me right in the centre of the town.

I often played between the trees and overgrown bushes running around wearing the surplice and flapping the sleeves in bird like reflection on the way back from a service. I thought it was a great game, flying in the dark of the winter's night.

This particular night in question I was jumping out of a bush and onto the path when I stopped absolutely dead in my tracks. I had landed inches in front of a large portly male who was a little, no more than a little, worse for the demon drink.

He stopped still in his unsteady tracks, gave a shout that rang out in the night, his eyes opened to what seemed the size of oranges then turned tail and ran shouting back down the path as if seeing a ghost. I still stood startled and rooted to the spot, then scampered off home not stopping for breath or to glance at any one. Who had frightened who the most?

Singing in church gave me a warm place to be in winter, a companionship where I was wanted and not ridiculed and more importantly the beginning of the sense of a higher being that did listen and understand my life difficulties.

I suppose around this time I gradually stopped talking to my imaginary animals and birds, replacing them with this all incarnate being, GOD. Saying that, my special friends still did make their appearances, but only when they felt necessary after Mother's aggressions.

Having attended Sunday school for most of the previous years I had an academic understanding of Him, his son Jesus and where they were to be found.

"Just close your eyes and see Him sitting on a cloud, in heaven," was the image given to all who attended. "If you need him just pray," so I did and He just stayed sat there on His cloud surrounded by angels. I even opened my eyes to look but he just sat there, smiling behind His white beard.

I was also famed at Sunday school for giving the wrong answer when quizzed about my father's name for the register. The elderly Sunday school mistress was compiling a list of parent's names, as given by the children. "What does your mummy call your daddy?" I was asked at a very tender age in front of the whole Sunday school. Quick as a flash I replied,

"The wife," this brought howls of laughter from the teacher and the other adults who relayed it back to mother when she came to pick me up. Needless to say I paid for my innocence and honesty when I got home.

Unfortunately it was a time when I needed something more realistic than this image of a man called GOD. A proper dad, you know, a real man who could deliver me from my life and place me with another family.

I had a proper dad, but he went away to leave me in a dysfunctional family. I needed a real family that has a dad, real pets, with lots of holidays away, and eats proper food; oh and with a garden that has a wood at the bottom.

A family that does not fight all the time or have a mother who rules with a fist of iron or belt of leather, was God going to deliver me this? No, but initially he did give me a sense of peace and beauty found only within His house.

St Peters is a large church built by rich Victorians who wanted to show off their wealth to all within this northern mill town. Sadly its style of delivery had reduced the congregation such that, by the late fifties, they almost rattled around inside the large worship area like peas in a drum. This fact did give each service a space and emptiness that made the parish church almost cathedral like inside.

In the West end of the church is a set of Stained Glass windows to rival any in buildings more famous than this. During evensong the setting sun would enhance the coloured glass and give the pictures and light a heavenly glow.

Such a beauty of colours and light I had never seen before on such a grand scale. This was God in all his glory. It gave me a feeling of peace that kept me in the choir long after my sell by date had passed for religion as an adolescent.

Never had I felt such a sense of peace and well being when life was so troubled for me. I watched the sun setting amongst the particles of coloured glass with awe ever time in spring and autumn. Summer months would give the window a glow that had resemblance of cool shade within the heat of the day. Winter meant that I was to watch and wait for His promise of brighter days to come. He had planted seeds of faith in me, through that window that would germinate and grow long after my life in Swinton had ended.

This Victorian monument built by the riches of capitalist profit acquired from the graft of the honest working classes, was actually portrayed as a glorification of peace and calm to me. The monetary aspect was beyond my comprehension as a child but the window was beautiful. Its colours and light fascinated me continually. The window still stands today, beauty personified.

24

The Juniors: Knobley and Dunce

Back to school now and my time in the junior's school at Moorside was no less traumatic than in the infants, just different. I can say in my favour that I was more ready for the hassle and well practiced in getting caned and standing outside of the classroom.

Streaming the pupils must have caused some consternation for the teaching staff when placing me appropriately. Never thick enough to be in the bottom set but naughty enough to be there. Was I to be placed with the no hopers?

My curse masked my intellect to deny me the top set ratings so I was eventually settled into the middle range of students, the 'W's. Top classes were called 'E' for excellent, Middle groups 'W' for workers and bottom set was labelled 'T' for triers. An educational branding system left behind, I hope, in the 21st century.

Initially on landing in the first year of this intermediate schooling I was mistakenly placed in the 'E's but that only lasted utill the first Christmas. It was with shame that I was downgraded to the 'W' class, a very rare occurrence. Talk of the year I was yet again, with more shame to contend with. Boy was I a natural born looser, welcome to the Juniors!

Again at this time I had bad days and not so bad days with my curse. I had missed so much of the basics in the infants that I was always playing catch up. I had a succession of teachers that used the cane with accuracy to 'enable' me to learn better or ensure I did not commit any more misdemeanours.

One particular such teacher was Mr Knobley. He was not a specifically violent or difficult man but he used his cane on me with regularity to instill in me the virtues of learning and to diminish the wickedness I pervaded.

The dress sense of the male teaching staff then was always a suit or tweed jacket often with brown brogue shoes. He also had the obligatory leather patches on his jacket and Mr Knobley always smelt of the same strong after shave.

Its odour was so strong that it was easily remembered but yet I have never smelt it since so have difficulty naming it. Perhaps one day someone somewhere will be wearing it and the perfume will send me right back to class 3W and that mans personal aroma.

I return to his cane, it was a polished piece of possibly

bamboo with a rounded stubbly end that rested on top of the blackboard in the wooden ridge. Its shiny knob just protruded above the moulding and was a constant reminder to me of the answer to any questions concerning any transgression. One particular incident in my memory bank was when we were learning to use the dictionary. How ironic for me, logical sequencing and alphabetic order were concepts always beyond my grasp, even today.

Ask my wife, Rachel, she knows my system for filing is leaving whatever out on view. If it gets tided away, then I can't see it and I've lost it forever. No logical sequencing in that.

Today we were to learn how to use a dictionary. I could understand Knobley's first instruction but could not keep up decoding the rest of the instructions about sequencing and lost the plot very early on in that particular lesson in question.

Fortunately to distract me I had various girl pupils around me. I could make faces at them and enjoy their reaction as their disgust spread across their faces. There was also the one directly in front who had her hair in tight pig tails in a Heidi fashion. The temptation to give those neat twists of brown hair a gentle tug was far too much in this time of dullness and boredom and intellectual blankness.

Reaching out across my desk I pulled one softly, enough to make it noticed but not aggressively enough to make the child cry or cry out in pain. I was soon spotted by the eagle like eyes of the class educator and brought to the front with a verbal reprimand that stilled the rest of the class. My right hand was extended for me and I soon felt the sharp sting that had resulted from the wood hitting my open palm with force and accuracy. I remember trying to hold back the tears and attempting to go back to my seat when his hand left mine.

These cameo pantomimes were always carried out in front of the watching audience, my class mates. As I turned towards my desk he shouted,

"Stewart, don't move, I've not done with you yet, stand still, just where you are and face the rest of the class."

This was a new venture from the classroom controller that I was not used to. Routine instilled in my behaviours the trek back to my seat or being sent outside to face the wall and, "Reflect upon what I had done wrong," but standing there, facing the class, I was soon to endure a new shaming a different ridicule. This pantomime was to gather momentum in front of its eager spectators and I was to play the part of Village Idiot to its optimum.

I stood at the front of the other children not knowing what Knobley was doing on his desk behind me. He asked me a question specifically based upon what I should have just learnt. "Name a word that would come just after five in the dictionary?" the middle aged educationalist asked. I can't remember exactly what I replied with, probably "six" or a word similar. No laughter from the watching peers. They had gathered the gravity of the situation I was in and dare not lighten it with an outburst of frivolity.

In my mind saying "six" was logical as I did not understand

the sequencing of letters in relationship to the alphabet.

Even today you can easily catch me out by asking what letter comes before any in the alphabet. I have to retort the whole list from 'A' right up to the one required then quickly go back one and give the right answer.

Knobley did not give me eye contact or a verbal reply; a silence fell across the square class room except for the noises the activity on the teacher's desk made. A large piece of grey card, used in the art session, was being folded and taped into a conical shape after a five letter word had been placed upon it in large capital letters.

"Go stand in the corner, Stewart," I was ordered and I knew I was not in any position to question his commanding authority. Our lot as 'pupils' was to receive, not to debate and discuss. We were recipients of education, not equals or given any parity in how it was distributed to us as pupils.

So I meekly walked over past his desk to the far corner at the front of the class. I stood looking at the corner expecting the class to resume their lesson. Knobley came up behind me and promptly explained to the class about some Dickensian novel where a character was sent to the corner and the Dunce's hat was placed on their head.

He told me to place one foot in the metal dustbin next to me and then I felt the cardboard cone being fitted into place on my head and the rest of the class laughing in hysterics. After a few seconds he shouted at them to quieten because it was no laughing matter when someone was the dunce of the class.

My fate was to stand for the rest of the day facing

the corner, hands clasped behind my back with a dunce's hat on, one foot in the class rubbish bin. The description placed in letters was so large that my class mates and all who passed on the corridor could see.

I do remember that uppermost in my mind I was more bothered about my mother finding out than the ridicule. I would be doubly punished for bringing shame upon her. How could she look the other mothers in the face if she saw them out shopping when they knew I had been so naughty and ridiculed so? Was someone from my class going to tell her? Were they to tell their parents at home who would dutifully pass the information over to mother when they saw her next? Or worse, was a letter to be sent home explaining my misdemeanour and being a written account enhancing the trouble it caused?

I dreaded my fate yet fate itself was to be kind to me that day. For some reason it was one of the few incidents at school mother never found out about. My punishment was to stay there within the establishment and not be doubled or repeated back at home.

This did not prevent me from living on tenterhooks for the next few days until I thought the issue had been fully ended and left at school. I had never heard the word Dunce before and wondered what it really meant, knowing it was demeaning but not sure how derogative. The part of it I did fully understand was the ridicule it gave me and the feelings of being absolutely inferior again.

I know now that I am not a dunce, I just learn differently. Written words had little meaning for me especially initially. My brain, through its miswiring, used to work very hard to convert them into something it understands. I learn, remember or see things though pictures, symbols or sensory elements, difficult in a society that used the written word as its main purveyor of information.

Pick up the old fifties children's novels on a car boot and count the pictures in them on one hand. Look at the wording, small tight heavy Times Roman script, a nightmare for me to decipher. Comic Sands is my easiest to read but again even today there is a campaign for 'clever people' to get rid of it. Is this possibly a last bastion of discrimination and handicapping for me to explain to others its wrongness?

It was especially difficult then for me to understand just words without the bank of years of learning and experiences to call upon that I have now acquired in life. I still have to remember names of things or people by association to another person or activity. I call them memory hooks.

The pure written or single spoken word holds no memory hooks for me, just fear of the unknown and a panic I have when under the pressure of having to remember them. It's like a fried egg sliding across the face of the Teflon coated pan, not stopping to become remembered. In fact words and snippets of information become more like scrambled eggs, all jumbled up, and not resembling its original form or context sliding across the Teflon aspects of my brain.

To this day I still struggle using a paper dictionary. Should I question myself with thoughts today such as, "Am I to still stand in society in corners with the dunce's hat on to tell all of my inadequacies and differences," or do I just accept the thing I cannot change or improve? Or is it not my issue but society's and those around me? Is this a debate on handicapping and disability to be used at another time, maybe?

Dunce I neither was nor am. I am just different, think differently and my brain works differently, miswired and not the norm but I am intelligent all the same.

How was Mr Knobley to know in those distant days about the brain and its many malfunctions? Had the term dyslexia been used or discovered then? Sometimes, I believe, teachers in those days were just people with a modicum of intellect, who had left the war to become apprentices alongside practicing professionals. With a basic list of qualifications and a year of this 'hands on' course for experience they were deemed qualified teachers. A balanced and learned way of working, maybe not?

Perhaps I had to suffer the consequences of this gap in broader understanding as probably did so many others historically. Or does lack of breadth of knowledge around child development, still happen today, surely not? This misfitting has given me a great empathy with others in situations that are similar to mine. People ridiculed because of their sexuality or skin colour. Their physical appearance or an intellectual disability may single them out and leave them open to mockery from uneducated people.

My training in empathy was a journey I suffered with and endured as a child. This left me as an adult with deep emotions about righting wrongs and standing up for others less blessed with skill and knowledge or aspects acceptable by the norm of society. I hope I wear truth and fairness as a cloak covering my actions in life.

Those people regarded in today's unbalanced and unfair society as lesser or inferior will always get my support and actions. Standing in a corner with a dunces hat on was just one episode of many that encouraged my inner mind and heart to truly believe in standing up for others, irrespective what the personal consequences of doing so could be.

These consequences that have dotted my life like black holes in space, causing me to run foul of many a one in authority over me or an unsympathetic system. Falling into the correct holes in society designed by others for us to fit into is not without pain for me, but it is a pain I can now gladly suffer so others can become acceptable as who they are. This pain is a good pain.

25

Piano Lessons and Being Late for the Blackley Visit

Around this time early in the Juniors I had tried piano lessons along with my brother. Mother just said to us both one day would we like to learn how to play an instrument and as there was an old stand up piano in the front room going to waste it seemed like the obvious choice.

Virtually all our relatives had a piano or some form of musical instrument played in their homes. Having a piano, poor as we were, seemed natural. Playing it was another conquest and I was never allowed to touch the old upright in the front room, well whilst Mother was around anyway.

Where Mother got the money from to pay for the lessons I will never know, perhaps on reflection her only brother may have sent up some from his home in Weybridge to cover such luxuries. Music was steeped into her side of the family and was seen as a young person's right to share in the melodic tone of some instrument or other.

Alan and I subsequently were sent off to a very strange man who lived with his parents, in a bungalow. It was a peculiar place, behind its metal spiked railings, yet the room with the piano in was eerily scary.

When the tutor came in I often had a peculiar feeling about him, I really did not like or relate to him. He taught piano to many children but I could never quite get the hang of the order the notes had to go in. He even tried to get me to remember the notes by using phrases like, "Every God Dog Deserves Favour." I remember the phrase but not the need or reasoning behind it.

"How silly!" I thought. Alan went at his lessons hell for leather and ended up an accomplished musician, backing many famous artists in his adolescent days as well as having his own band and touring Europe.

My relationship with playing music did not relate through the piano forte or this man that I never felt at ease with. The sooner I was out of this situation the better for me! I was a tickled trout on the river bank flapping about, gasping for air, wanting to return to where I was more comfortable. I just could not be bothered with the fight to learn and gave up interest not too long after starting especially after being late one notorious day.

I was not late for the piano lessons but coming home on my old Raleigh bike I decided to stop on the Clough and play for a while and I ended up being late for mother's trip across Manchester to see her sister.

Time stood still on the Clough for me whenever I was

there playing. That particular day I had a great adventure playing Ivanhoe then hunting for frogs and wild life. Unfortunately mother had planned to visit her sister straight after I should have arrived back at lunch. She had told me to get home as quickly as I could so I could be ready for the long trip across Manchester on two buses.

I had forgotten, easily done, it's a skill I still use to perfection and without any effort today, good old short term memory loss. It's a classic for getting me into scrapes even now. Forgetting things, especially if I have just been told them and it's a long list of more than two items, is a constant issue. Can you imagine how you feel, as an adult, when someone has just asked you to do something and you then ask them to repeat it because you can only remember the first part? This has driven people close to me mad over the years.

Fortunately nowadays Rachel understands and she just kindly passes it off and repeats herself. Back then it would lead to many naggings with mother and disciplinary actions at school. That day was no exception. My curse had kicked in and I was to pay for it.

I had blissfully played on after my piano lesson without caring for anyone or anything. A shout brought me back to reality. "Christopher, come here!" I spun around to see Mother's scrawny outline on the horizon at the top of the gully. Why is she here I thought. My blood ran cold and I knew I was in trouble.

It was so unreal to see mother here, on the Clough. This was my world and she never, ever came into it. I felt sick deep down inside. "Get up here now you little swine, had you forgotten we are all going out to Aunties this afternoon?"

In those days communication between the families was via letters, no-one had telephones except Uncle in Weybridge. So to be able to tell my Aunty in Blackley that we were to be late was a practical impossibility. This fact only exasperated the situation for me. Today a quick text message would have put the situation right, not so in those days.

I scrambled up the sandy slope and was greeted by one of mothers rasping right hand slaps across my face. "We should have left here ages ago," she screamed. "You little bastard, your lesson finished hours ago, what have you been doing?" her scream was high pitched. I knew we were alone on the Clough. If there were others around her she would have been more discrete with her behaviour, suppressing her anger and hiding her cruelty.

Mother hit and blasted me with insults and questions all the way home. Her anger remained unabated. I remember washing in the bathroom and changing into clean clothes with her close attention and constant physical prompts. She was real angry and vented it at me with full force.

Alan and Margaret were sat on the couch downstairs, been ready to go for ages, and in great fear of her. They did not move, petrified that one movement out of line meant they would get the nagging and smacking I was soaking up. I had not meant to do it, really, I just forgot.

Forgetting is a trait of mine and is almost like having dementia for all my life. In adulthood I have been assessed

Piano Lessons and Being Late for the Blackley Visit

by a psychologist who was a Dyslexia specialist, for my short term memory loss and it is pretty naff. I need repetition or 'hooks' to be able to remember even the simplest list of things. Any list of tasks or verbal information is nearly impossible for me to retain.

This professional opinion of hers would have meant nothing back then. I had made mother late for a visit to her sisters and I was to pay for it. I knew the pressure she was to put me under would last a long time, all day in fact. Only easing off the pedal whilst we were travelling to our Aunty on the bus and in front of my Aunt where I could breathe a little better knowing I could not be hit or nagged.

I was told I had to stop crying as we walked through the estate and towards our cousin's door. Don't get me wrong I loved going to see relatives and when they visited us it was another fun day, respite from her issues. We would play for hours in Boggat Hole Clough just behind their house on the White Moss Estate. I could read their comics, play with their toys and eat a real spread for tea.

On trips to our house I recall one specific day in particular when we had gone out to Dean's Park. The session on the swings and slide was cut short by my mistaking a footing on the big slide and I came down head over buttock. This fall gave me more than just a few cuts and I'm not sure if concussion was also on my agenda. Anyway I was dragged home to curtail the discussions between sisters and soundly beaten after they had gone up to the Town Hall for the 57 bus home.

178

Another occasion etched in to my happy family memory box was when both Mother and Aunty took us all to Worsley, a posh village down the road. We played in the woods for ages and ended up with forty shades of dirt all over us. Strangely as Aunty thought it was OK and just what kids did there was no great reprimand.

We just all ended up in one bath together, yes five lads and one girl. A touch of washing up liquid and the bath was full of foam. All in the bath together was on the pretext of using one lot of hot water but I'm sure it would not have been allowed in today's society. We all just thought it was fun!

Before we all met up on this particular day mother's instruction to me was not to play out with my cousins but stay in her eye range all the time we were there. How quiet I must have been that day. All the time I was there I knew I was to get more of the same as we went home and then before I got to bed. The pressure of this fear was real for Alan, Margaret and I. We must have had a certain quality mentally that enabled us to survive such an onslaught. This was a learnt quality, learnt through hours and years of endless conflicts with mother.

Back to the piano lessons needless to say, by mutual consent, I gave them up very shortly after this particular episode. Out of disaster often come respite and a better way forward. Well almost!

26

Dr Smith and a Claim to Fame

Mother also did try, somewhat unknowingly, to cure me of my curse. Sometime after starting junior school and giving up piano lessons she took me to see Dr Smith our family GP.

He was a very mild mannered man who lived in an extremely large Victorian house cum surgery in Eccles. An ex Army colleague of my dad, but of much higher rank than Dad, we still went to him after Dad had left because Dr Smith was such a gentleman. His mind and attitudes were not corrupted by the ravages and horrors of the war all men of his age had gone through.

He was at his old wooden roll top desk when we went in, the room had a wax polish smell unless it was tea time and the smell of a stew or meat cooking wafted into the surgery from his kitchen just at the back of his surgery.

He leaned over towards me and smiled. "Now young Christopher what is the matter?" Mother sat me next to him and started to complain about my 'psychomotor' skills or lack of them.

"He's always sick on the bus, we have to sit him next to the open door wherever we go or he will just throw up his dinner. He can't go on swings and he's always falling over his feet." The list continued in front of me, "He knocked a glass pane out of the front room cabinet last week," she complained.

If the truth were to be known it was this tripping up and putting my hand through the glass that was the last straw and prompted her to drag me for a medical consultation. The list extended."He falls down stairs and can't go up any heights. What am I going to do with him Dr Smith?" she asked.

The left-handedness and poor English skills were not connected in those days to lack of balance, my clumsiness and a brain miswiring. How medical science and educational psychology has improved today!

Dr Smith turned back to me and asked in his soft posh accent unheard of in my everyday life: "How do you feel about this Christopher?" I cannot remember my answer but do recall him asking and I felt nervous! Such answers to questions were always left to Mother.

Now in a nineteen fifties medical and educational system, all the behaviours that I displayed were collectively a curse. Today it can still haunt me but there is much more understanding and empathy around dyslexia to support me.

Dr Smith and a Claim to Fame

This kind and gentle medical practitioner gave me a warmed handed examination. He looked thoroughly into my ears, eyes and up my nose then at the rear of my throat. He asked me questions about my sporting skills, my favourite football team, tried to unbalance me by pushing my shoulders with his hand and finally had me catching a ball.

After some solemn contemplation he declared to my mother, "Christopher will need his tonsils and adenoids out as well as his sinuses flushing through, other than that I can only suggest he goes to dancing school, which will improve his balance!" My trip to hospital is duly recorded elsewhere in this book. How medical science and educational psychology has further improved today!

Mother promptly took me to the dancing school my younger sister went to on the way home in Eccles. Without the handiness of your own transport often things were done 'while you were there' or in line with bus timetables. That visit was to lay foundations for an aspect of life that I could only have dreamt of as such a little boy.

Little did Dr Smith know that my days at the Shelia Payant Dance Academy would stand me in good stead and give me confidence boosting roles in society later in my life? I gained a wider skill range needed to hold down a more normal life through my stage experiences than I probably did at any school I attended.

This was an unintentional positive action that mother must take the acclamation for amidst her legacy of cruelty and instability. This was to be a step into the real world

182

of fantasy that was, in its entirety, acceptable to the rest of society and in fact enabled me with some minor talent to give joy and happiness to others. A rare gift but one I later took with both hands (and feet!) and demonstrated a small town expertise that also gave me small town fame.

I soon started attending the dancing school along with my sister Margaret who already went. Now for a young boy in working class Salford in the late nineteen fifties dancing was not an open option so I had to keep quiet at school and in my neighbourhood about my private life.

To be fair I was quite polished at this following Mothers influence on my life. I was used to having a vivid imagination so living a double life was not as difficult for me as maybe other more normal children would find it. Ballet, Tap and Stage Dancing was not a pass time I fell naturally or easily into.

In fact basically I had great difficulty coordinating my limbs with my brain, even when it had the support of music. Irrespective of that difficulty, the whole experience did eventually leave me with a legacy of both a sense of rhythm and stage presence, both to become useful in later life.

The former I was to enjoy and use on many social occasions. The latter came into to use later making some money entertaining people and further on in my professional life teaching and entertaining young people with severe learning difficulties.

Unfortunately my short term memory loss meant that I could never remember easily sequences in the dance routines set out for me. One particular show we did as a dancing school I went on stage to do my tap solo to the tune 'Forty Second Street' and completely forgot virtually every step. The whole practice and rehearsed sequence was not to be recalled as it should have been in the foot lights.

Poor Shelia Payant, the Dancing School Owner, stood in the wings watching, she was so astonished at my antics. When I came off stage she told me that she could not understand where that new routine came from but was just glad my feet kept tapping throughout the number. I just busked the whole three minutes and made up the tap dance as I went along.

This was a skill I was to hone into almost perfection with my mouth as I grew older, busking my way out of trouble and filling in spontaneously. Forgetting what I was supposed to do and covering my inadequacies with quick fire answers comes very naturally to me now but in those days I struggled.

Doing it with my feet was even harder. I often put myself into the position of great stress by going on stage in competitions and shows trying to remember complex sequences. It was a far greater stress when I danced with others. They always remember where they were supposed to be and what to do. I often just pranced around in a world of my own desperately trying to remember a 'hook' in the music or movements to get back into the sequence with.

Like an actor learns lines I was expected to remember things abstract to my natural way of thinking or doing.

Mission Impossible but upon reflection, good fun, maybe some of the audience smiled?

Coupled to this was the fact that I was not the most natural mover with my body, my clumsiness was exasperated in the glare of the stage lights slap bang in front of an audience. I knew I would never get anywhere with my dancing but it did get me out of the house and often it would gain me that feeling the applause gives you deep inside.

The thrill of working on an audience, getting them into the palms of your hands and then the glow you get when they give you their spontaneously warm and appreciative applause through their clapping is an excitement immeasurable. Despite my ham footed efforts over the next few years the smell of the grease paint and the glow from the applause did give me a wonderful feeling of excitement and self worth.

This started to balance the other aspects of life that held me back and get me suppressed. It was of great value to me living the secret life of a dancer to gain this adoration, however fleeting and it so contrasted from the other deep dark times in my life at that time. This time also gave me my first claim to fame as a child.

Towards the end of my time in Junior School, or it could even have been early secondary school, the lady who ran the dancing school duly informed my mother that two film producers were visiting the Wendover Hotel at Monton Green and interviewing boys with stage experience for a film they were making. She requested that I and the only other lad in the school, my friend Perzo, attend and gave us the time and date.

Perzo's family was originally from Hungary and came over in the brief revolution in 1956. He was naturally talented at dancing and good looking to boot, a couple of years younger than me, but a real friend.

I was duly scrubbed and had my best clothes on. We both entered the room without our parents where two older men were sat at a round table with lots of paperwork on the white table cloth. One asked Perzo and I various questions about our stage experiences.

I was asked to read a short paragraph from a story. The other one then questioned me about the Manchester United team and who I would like to play like. I told him the goal keeper, Harry Greg. Strange situation this was for me and I felt I was on the edge of another world that was so far removed from my little life.

Towards the end of the interview they told us both that we were a little too young and small for whom they were looking for in their film and wished us both well. I told my mother outside and then one of the men then came to see her and explained why we were unsuitable.

A lot later it transpired that they were making a number of films, one of which eventually was 'Kes' and unknown to me I had just been auditioned for a major part. Now every time I watch the film I wonder what would have happened to me if I had fitted the bill. Would I have led another life different to the one I now have as my history? Perhaps but I would not have been sat here at my computer trying hard to write my story for you to read.

Experiences I had are not better or worse, just different with consequences that are different. No 'If only' with me, just 'different' and I only dream about my future now not my past. Still I was not offered the chance of working with a real live bird of prey, Kes. That was a chance I sadly missed!

The time spent at dancing school had engrained into me some sense of rhythm and my coordination did get better. My many years of struggle to perform eloquently with my body were to pay dividends later on when following a short break in Amateur Dramatics I took to the road as a mobile DJ in Manchester. A tale to be told at another time!

27

Mother Leaving Us

Remember the old adage, "What doesn't kill you makes you stronger?" This next episode of our sad early life might fall deep into that category but I'm not sure how much stronger it made me.

Mother's instability intensified after Dad left and her playing her mind games on us did not relent either when we were small children or as we were growing up in her care. I wonder if she knew how devastating it was for us to receive those onslaughts as she tried to make us behave or beat the devil out of me. Maybe she felt it was the only way to control the three children she had under her power.

Only once did she take her anger outside of the house into such a public place where the rest of the world could see and hear her behaviour. The night in question was when she said she had had enough of us all, even Margaret.

What specific incident had triggered this particular chapter of humiliation and degradation, my memory does not recall. I just remember the consequences of her strategy to correct us.

She had decided to leave us and had packed her suitcase in front of her desperate, crying children during this particular episode of nagging as if to emphasise any trauma she could impart. Remember, I would be around seven or eight at the time, Alan eleven and Margaret only about four.

It was winter and a very dark night. She was adamant she was leaving us to our own devices and that it would stop us all from being so naughty. She had screamed at us for ages, told us all we just were not worth living for, then slammed the front door hard and was gone!

The house stood briefly silent apart from our soft sobbing. What were we to do here left all alone without her to feed us or look after us; we had no money and little food in the house? Alan quickly told both Margaret and I to get our coats on and we would follow her. It was the only answer.

All three of us all trooped out holding hands into the dark and caught a glimpse of her through our tears, turning at the bottom of the drive towards the rear of the bus sheds. We followed through the dim lamp lit streets sobbing and trying to catch up with her.

The very streets that Lowry walked collecting his rents, before painting them and becoming famous were now providing the back drop for this tiny drama in the insignificant lives of three children and their deranged mother.

Why, after all the beatings we had taken from her, did we try so hard to get her back into our lives I'll never know? We managed to catch her up only to be greeted with a deluge of abuse. We were the reason she had to leave; we were the cause of her to feel so bad about herself. We were the children from the devil and we should go back to hell. She repeatedly told us this in an uncompromising way, oblivious to the other people who occasionally passed by giving this strange group of night travellers a second look.

"Why," she kept shouting at us, "Why were we the way we were?" She had done all she could to bring us up properly on her own. "I just want to kill myself and that will get me away from you bloody lot," she screamed at us.

We trudged on, crying through the dingy town that night only a few footsteps behind her, stopping only when Mother turned around to throw her torrent of abuse at us. The orange glow from the streetlights and the shadows playing on her face in the dark night gave her a distinctive look, almost witch like.

This episode was different from the others. We felt very unsafe out here, on the streets. It was a new and frightening change to her behaviour, where would this night end? We just walked in the dark, sobbing and offering our heart rendering apologies, following her and having to endure the words of vilification.

Certainly Alan and I tried to counter her behaviour. Margaret just followed, her emotions caught up with the situation but not fully understanding the gravity of Mother's actions. This was also her first time facing the rages Mother doled out to Alan and I on a regular basis.

Mother knew how to hurt us, both bodily and deep inside. She knew how to send us to the brink of despair and how to mentally beat us into non human beings, without any rights or future. Mother gave us such strong feelings of guilt and shame, for just being ourselves.

We walked for ages until she finally stopped and turned around on us. "I'll come back," her anger was not concealed in her voice. "I'll come back if you little bastards can change your ways and be good." A list of wrongdoing then issued from her lips aimed like flaming arrows into our inner selves.

It worked, we had all begged her to return amid our tears and we told her we would have life changing behaviour. She turned back and we yet again trundled behind her in a very belittling shuffle. Her venom was still spitting from her mouth, each sentence cutting into us and leaving salt on each verbal wound.

That night back in the house we went up to bed very quietly. An eerie calm had descended upon our house in Stonegate drive. Mother must have been tired from all her ranting and running around the town.

We went to sleep that evening not quite knowing what the next day held for us. Was she to be there or would she have gone into the night, never to be seen again? Strangely life as we knew got back to normality in its bizarre little way. Perhaps that was all we could cope with as a family or as tired individuals. She did not kill herself nor did we put an end either to ourselves or her, so as children our insignificant little lives just went on.

Gradually the exceptionally good behaviour from me started to crumble and within a few weeks I was right back to the square that I was always in with her caused by my behaviour, followed by one of her beatings.

A little later on we did have another strange episode where mother disappeared for a while in circumstances us children had no information about or explanation for. We did have a precursor to her disappearance but as children we were never aware enough to read the signs.

I remember that we all walked down Worsley road to a Social Services home in silence that particular afternoon. Mother did not speak, just walked along side us. She had told us all to get our best clothes on and have a good wash. We were going out with her and had to be very good. I would never ask where we were going or question things. Time and Mother's behaviour had taught me never to put any form of conflict into a situation, no matter how good the circumstances were.

We soon entered the newly built office style building and sat in a small reception area. I remember little as at the time I felt that I was of no consequence there. Mother spoke to another woman in a small side office and came out still saying nothing.

It was the only time I went to that building not realising mother was trying to place us somewhere for a few months. Later in my youth I recognised the building as possibly a

Social Services Care Home for Children. On reflection as adults, why we were to be sent away is a mystery to us children even today and a point of speculation whenever we meet together. We did get split up and sent away for at least a few months but it was family and friends who came to the rescue of this rag taggle band of infants, not the authorities.

28

Living with Aunty Julian in Denton

Very soon after the Care Home visit we were separated as a family and transported across Manchester to various family and friends for a few months. Alan was bundled off to Aunty Alice's in Stockport, Margaret went to live with our Aunty in north Manchester and I ended up in Denton at Aunty Julian's.

Apparently none of mother's blood relative wanted to house me for an unspecific time period so her very old friend from school days took me in for however long I was to be there. Aunty Julian was the only one who had the time or space for me it seemed.

Denton is on the east side of Manchester and I had visited this kind couple often before. Uncle John and Aunty Julian were the epitome of what caring parents were supposed to be. She was warm and loving, he quiet, fair in his judgments and had a gentle but strong way about him.

Visiting meant another very long bus ride, going through Piccadilly Gardens in the centre of town, through Ardwick and past Belle Vue towards the Pennines. One bus that had a terminus both near her home and our house. Surely this was an omen that I had to be there? This journey was always exciting for me, just to pass through this magical place of Belle Vue looking out over the upstairs to see its enchanted spaces.

Belle Vue was the fairground and zoo in Manchester in its day and is now long closed. It held the speedway track, a large concert hall and many caged exotic animals.

My occasional visits left me with memories that brought some of my fantasies into reality. I had actually ridden an elephant in there, yes a real live elephant! To the best of my memory this poor old beast had two benches strapped to each side and it had to stand between two long high walkways for visitors to clamber aboard on to its side. I had cajoled mother to let me ride it and the thrill of that short journey still stays with me today.

Belle Vue also gave me the insight of real wildlife when I saw the lions and tigers close up. These infrequent visits fuelled my imagination, I felt as if I had been given the Ok to fanaticise because I had seen the real wild animals, smelt them and seen them moving right before my eyes.

The smell of the lion's cages, the height of the giraffes and the sound of the seals barking were etched into the brain to be recalled later when on safari in Wardley woods. I could now stalk them in the woods and shoot at them with my imaginary double barrel shot gun from the top of my elephant.

In some ways such a wild fantasy was not too far from the truth. Somewhere in Worsley woods, which was adjacent to Wardley woods, there is an elephant's grave, well hidden, that I use to seek out and visit. Folklore tells that this large mound of earth was the final resting home of a travelling circus elephant in Victorian times that had extinguished its life whilst visiting the locality. It had been buried in the woods and only the mound of earth was left as a reminder of this majestic beast.

I use to dream of it rising in the night from its grave to wander around our local woodlands looking for its real home. I would imagine I could hear it trumpeting in the distance. I could call it, just like Mahout, the Elephant boy and it would come to me. I would track through the undergrowth with the elephant behind me, holding its trunk gently on my shoulder whilst I found the way to the East Lancs road. We would then ride together along the new road to Liverpool where I could get it aboard a ship going to India and home for the beast.

The elephant was a far cry from the only real animals I had. Not really allowed to have pets one summer I found an old suitcase and punched holes through the top then placed grass and a saucer of water in it. On my many travels to the Clough and woods that summer I collected several frogs and toads, carrying them home especially carefully in my pockets. On arrival at Stonegate Drive I would gently place them into the suitcase which I hid away from mother's knowledge under the old Anderson Shelter converted to a shed. These would be my pets and I would visit them before I rode out to play each day.

Slugs and snails were collected by me to feed them on and I thought I was being ever so kind. Little did I realise at that time that wildlife needs a freedom to survive. Life in any small enclosure is not right and against all the laws of nature. Sure enough they did not survive the summer and I gave up trying to keep and breed amphibians as pets in such a small space.

Back in Denton, Aunty Julian had three children of her own, the youngest just older than me. I was to share a bedroom with her two lads, Ian and Simon and sleep on the floor under an eiderdown. Continental quilts had not been invented then for the masses. I was fortunate that it was in the spring and summer time so I did not need to be kept to warm.

The middle bedroom in the large terraced house was just above the back living room so the heat from the coal hearth would take the chill off the bedroom anyway.

Both of her boys were my heroes, and what I really wanted my brothers to be like them. Perhaps in reality if they had to live under such an evil mother then they would have behaved just like Alan and I did.

This was to be a great 'holiday' for me and lasted many months. Just sleeping on the floor was an adventure. I would drift into the land of nod pretending I was on a ship travelling to foreign lands or in the Army on manoeuvres awaiting the call to battle, ready at any time. Sleeping on the floor was as near to sleeping outside for me as I could get at the time.

Whilst staying there I went to the same primary school as Simon and did not suffer any of the aggravations I had at my own school, Moorside. Maybe because I was only a temporary pupil or it was a softer regime in the school I don't know but it enabled me to see what school should be like. I was welcomed and never caned. This was dreamland for me. On the down side I felt more of the pressure when I returned back to my old school from this enforced break, having tasted a warmer and more empathic learning establishment.

There were actually only a couple of minor negative incidents to the Denton visit but considering my lifestyle they were of little consequence in the whole scheme of things. One was at the beginning of the stay, the other after I returned to Swinton.

On the first night at Laburnum Road straight after tea Aunty Julian informed me that I would need a bath. Maybe I was six or seven I cannot recall exactly but imagine my horror when I realised she was to bath me. Don't get me wrong, I loved my Aunty Julian but to have a woman bath me was well, just not on at that age.

Why she wanted to I can only speculate today at her intention. Maybe she was looking for marks on my body? I'm not sure but knowing her she would only have my best interest at heart.

What mother's family and friends knew of our situation we did not know at the time. Aunty in Blackley only realised mother smoked when she fell ill with cancer in the last months of her life. This aunt was not in any great financial condition to support mother in her monetary plight of bringing up us three on the little dad sent as maintenance.

Both Aunt and Uncle had often bought material to give to mother to make clothes with for us both and most of Margaret's dancing costumes were made from material gifts from Uncle John and our beloved Aunty. They also would bring food on their many visits to help supplement our diet with.

Imagine her horror when her sister found out mother had been spending her money on cigarettes and secretly at that! To hide such a secret carefully for so long may mean that her sisters or friends did not know of all the tribulations going on at Stonegate Drive. Surly though they must have been suspicious?

Later in life Aunty in Blackley once told me of the time that we visited her and she saw Margaret take a slice of bread. Please remember food in our house was strictly rationed by mother and not because of the aftermath of the war. The table at Auntie's was set with a feast, a quality and quantity of food commonplace when we visited relatives, yet never on our daily agenda at home.

Margaret had apparently looked around the room to see if anyone was looking and had taken a slice of white bread, cut corner to corner as happened when visitors arrived. She then ate it as if it was the last piece on earth. This episode had shocked Aunty Amy and although she never mentioned it to Mother or Margaret, she told me later that because of that she had began to wonder what was going on at Stonegate Drive as we grew up.

Back in Denton Aunty Julian watched as I stood in her bathroom with the hot water run and the room steaming up. We never had hot, full baths at home so this was to be yet another luxury, but the cost for me was for Aunt Julian to see my private parts!

I had got down to my underpants in front of her. She tried to reassure me in her gentle way of talking, relating my situation to her two boys. "Now Christopher, you've just got the just the same as Simon and Ian you know," I recall her saying.

"Well not really," came my rapid reply, "Ian has a new bike and Simon has got a telescope, I've only got an old bike with metal wired brakes that Alan had a few Christmas ago." She fell about laughing at me.

In all innocence I had replied to her statement, which I thought had sidetracked me from thinking about her seeing my private parts. "Oh Christopher. I'll just let you get on with it and wait outside if you need any help," she did love me and let me know it.

I had never had such a gentle mother figure in my life before, and it endeared me to her forever. Uncle was just as sweet but with a masculine strength. He was a fitter at Metal Box and very clever with his hands, making and repairing all manner of things in his shed up the garden.

He had constructed a beautiful wooden fitted kitchen in their large terraced house well before the onset of Ikea or MFI. I had not seen such a kitchen before and would often wonder at it, opening doors and draws feeling them swing or slide with the ease only a craftsman can give to such natural material. He also had a garden beyond the back gate and spent many hours with me digging, potting and getting his beloved Dahlias to show their beauty in all their glory.

Today I still have a fondness for Dahlias and have just taken cuttings in the greenhouse this very morning ready to transfer them to an outdoor bed. I now have a love of growing and propagating.

Going back home after the stay at Aunty's I took over a small patch of ground in the garden and practiced growing things such as cuttings from other plants. With no one on hand to guide me or show me the skills needed I floundered on my own but the passion for growing plants stayed with me all my life. Remember, skills passed on in love are rarely forgotten.

Another wonder at Denton for me that was Aunty Julian had a cat, named Frisky. Not so frisky now as age had caught up with her, so I would be able to sit next to it and stroke the soft fur as she sat akin the fire in the back room.

You see I had never had a real pet that lived in the house, so here was the actual, real thing, right here for me to stroke and help feed, a real live cat. The thrill of having an actual animal to pet helped me in the journey of laying all my fantasy animals to rest. Today I am blessed with a wife who adores cats and we have ten of them, all individual and all loved.

Living with Aunty Julian in Denton

What a time I had in Denton. The cat, good food, no nagging or beatings, a school that treated me like a real person, Simon's telescope in my bedroom, hot baths that were filled to the top and the love of two kind people who wanted to spend their time with me.

I was also a party to using the telescope and viewing the stars close up. I remember wondering if God had seen me looking at Him. Was he just past the moon I wondered? Whatever the reason for this enforced break was I did not know or care at the time. I was being given a glimpse of real family life as I wanted it to be and as it should be for all children growing up. If I never saw my mother again I would not have cared or cried.

The other negative side at the end of this bliss was returning to mother and that house where life for me just picked up where it left off. Yet I had been given a taste, the shortest, sweetest glimpse, of how life for me should have been. Was it now more cruel for me because I had seen the Promised Land and been refused a permanent visa?

Only the thoughts of holidays on my bike, away from her in those fields and woods kept me sane, hanging on to a fantasy world far removed from reality. That was my way of getting me through the reality that was my living hell.

29

Swinton Baths

As my age began to get towards double figures I was allowed to journey across Swinton on my own more and to spend time in such places as the great hundred year old baths that stood in Victoria Park. They were initially dedicated as a monument for the working classes to keep clean and learn how to swim yet heralded a new chapter for me in growing up.

I would visit the baths on a summer's day with a very begrudging brother. It cost Sixpence to get in and thruppence for a Bovril. This was the price of another rare escape from the reality of Mother's regime.

It was to me a very large red shiny brick building with a grand entrance and a large glass roof. On the journey towards the citadel one could hear the screams and shouts of other young people enjoying the wet play. These sounds were amplified because of the tiled interior and spread for quite a distance beyond the railings that surrounded the building.

Males were split from females directly after entering as was the want of our moralistic Victorian ancestors. After changing behind the metal doors of the cubicles that had the edges aged with rust we would take the measured barefoot walk to a large shower.

This was the place where I first saw pubic hair as men occasionally showered in their birthday suits and little boys cowered to cover their own bits and embarrassment with giggles. A quick walk through the freezing footpool, then gasping at the warmth as you went into the vast tiled area that held the depths of clean water.

I would not jump straight into the water. I would engage with the melee of echoing noise and the chlorine smelling atmosphere. I would then stop at the top of the large steps down the shallow side that beckoned you in.

It was cold, especially after the hot shower that relinquished you of the world's dirt. Cold enough to get you to take time to acclimatise but the thrill and excitement of swimming around soon made you feel you could stay forever.

Tatty in comparison to modern day bathing areas Swinton Baths was unrivalled in its treasurers then on a hot day to play and swim in. Safe, clean and far enough away to give you nearly a full days entertainment which included the walk there and back through the dirty old streets of Victorian Swinton.

30

The Canyon in Wardley Woods

You will have gathered that I spent much of my time going home from school via the Clough or playing on the Indoos. As I grew my range during the school holidays expanded to the slightly more distant play areas of Wardley and Worsley woods.

How ancient the woodlands are I really don't know but there I was to almost live a second life, relinquishing the pain and fear that ruled at home. It was freedom for me and as long as I was back for supper time my bottle of water and a few slices of bread were sufficient sustenance. Summers and good weather brought about my release from her and any time spent directly under her power.

A short cycle ride up the East Lancs Road and I entered into my pleasure land. Some days I would dismount along the cycle path just before the Tyldsley loop rail track and wait for coal wagons to pass pulled by short steam tank engines. I would then enter the wooded area, a jungle of adventure that was mine and mine only, except, of course when others from the area happened to be there. Some days I would be covered up in the undergrowth and watch them as they played around the Canyon. Other days I would join them in their adventures.

The Canyon was special space in the centre of the woods with less tree cover but great in resources for activities. A stream ran down one side and a massive tree grew alongside it. Its waters had, over a period of time, carved a large gully into the soft sandy soil creating a steep sided canyon.

The depth of the canyon must have been 20-30 feet and one strong branch from the large tree hung over it like an outstretched arm willing the action minded to place a rope swing from it. Nature could not have given so many youngsters from the locality so much pleasure and not some little pain usually caused by the Canyon Swing.

A large rope almost always hung from the tree's arm and with a run and accurate jump I could launch myself across the gully and stream into space. The rope was never long enough to reach the other side but the sensation of flying through mid-air was just fantastic and tested most of my vesicular sense to its extreme.

The thrill of being suspended in motion so high above terra firma was exhilarating, even though it made me so dizzy so quickly. If I did not judge my return to the banking correctly I would often land backwards, causing myself some pain and a lot of dirt to inhabit my legs and clothes. Sometimes Alan and his mates would go there to test themselves against nature on the Canyon Swing.

One particular time I was party to playing with them and some other lads all taking turns to try to go as far out as possible. The different delivery of style was incredible amongst the budding space travellers. Some were holding on to the small piece of wood placed at the bottom of the rope as a makeshift seat in twos. Some were running from take off at an angle to the stream and twisting around as they flew effortless into the thin air. Showing off I would call it!

A halt was called to the proceedings by one of the gang and he suggested we try to see how many can swing out from the bank together. A recipe for excitement and thrills not without its dangers but dangers lost on such excited young males!

The group of apprentice gravity defying youths started to swing out across the ravine, first two then three adding another body to the weight of the pendulum each time it approached the near banking. I can remember I was about sixth and by the time another two were added my arms were aching from the weight of other bodies held against me.

Getting this mass of children out across the ravine was becoming more and more difficult. With one almighty push from the gang left on the bank the overweighted rope swung out to the sound of the children's screams of excitement.

The Canyon in Wardley Woods

There is nothing more inevitable than the inevitable but as a child you never know that or even necessarily learn from it. The tree and branch bowed with the weight and then a snap was heard throughout the woods. It drowned the screams of us all out for a few seconds as the old rope could take no more. The bindings snapped halfway down from the branch to the wood to which we were all clinging.

Right over the middle of the stream, with its human cargo as high from the ground as they could possibly be, we were dragged down into the stream. Our fall was cushioned only by the couple of inches of water running below us and the soft sand that the dirty water ran over and each other's bodies.

I felt the pain in my arm as it took the full force of both my own and someone else's weight. Others had fallen on their feet and some upside down. We must have looked a very sorry sight. The group had instantly gone from brave buccaneers to sad, wet, hurt children in the time it took to fall 20 or so feet.

One lad broke his glasses and I was in such a way that I could not ride my faithful old blue bike home but had to suffer the indignity of walking back covered in mud and with wet shorts on.

I recovered a day or so later, hiding the adventure from mother by landing home when she was not in and withdrawing up to our bedroom. My leg stopped hurting the next day and it was a small price to pay for such an extreme testing of nature against the thrill of the ride. The swing had been pushed beyond its limits and had not survived. When it was replaced we treated it with a little more respect.

The dapple shaded locale around the Canyon Swing also held a short cycle track area. Its micro geography was such that from a large flat circular area high up, called the pit stop, there was a wide path that went down an almost vertical drop for 10 feet, alongside the stream to flatten out onto a circuit run. This run went in a large oval, around several trees, rising up at the far end only to turn back upon its self and go up a steep hill to return to the flat area opposite the start.

It made a perfect cycle racetrack, wide enough to take four bikes each race and bendy and hilly enough to test a competent rider. Small gangs of kids would meet there and set up races between themselves. There was always time to admire each other bikes and stare in wonder at a real tracker with a 'fixed wheel', the height of 'street cred' in its day, long before BMX or Mountain bikes were ideas on the designers paper.

We would self-police the races having age or using bike sizes to elicit some form of handicapping. Again the sun shone brightly this particular hot summer's day and we welcomed playing under the dapple shade the mature trees offered.

I parked my old metal-braked Phillips bike up on the flat pit stop ground and placed my water and bread under it to watch the racing. My bike was no match for any other there but it was mine and I did clean and oil it with a regularity that made it as fast as it could mechanically be.

209

The Canyon in Wardley Woods

If only my thin little legs could grow to provide something like decent muscle power!

The whole pit stop was buzzing with kids and bikes. There was a gang of lads from another area, Alan and his mates and two or three others I think, so there was quite a gathering. No trouble between us all because we sort of knew each other or at least someone knew someone else from the other gang.

Who's bright idea to have an all comers race I don't remember but they must be held to account when they go up to the pearly gates and St Peter asks them of their sins on earth. We all instantly and naively decided it was a great idea.

The smallest were to go to the front largest at the rear. All of us were to attempt ten laps, the winner being first back to the top after ten goes around. I was promptly placed right at the front with two others alongside me and all the rest filled in behind across the top flat area.

It was to be the race of all races here at the Canyon Swing. The thrill of having the twenty-foot drop into the stream alongside the left hand edge only added to the excitement. Someone shouted "1-2-3 Go!" and we all set off, hell for leather, as if our lives depended upon coming in first.

There must have been twelve or thirteen budding scramblers setting off down that first slope. The damp woodland air whistled past my face as I tried to remain at the front against larger cycles and more skilllful riders. How long was this test of youth, courage and skill to actually last?

My judgment on passing the first protruding tree root was inadequate and I hit it, only to continue my movement forward but without my bike. The front wheel had stopped against the hard twisted wood and the rear wheel just went up and over the rest of the bike in its momentum forward. I flew into the air losing my grip on the handlebars and was tossed over the front wheel. This act on its own was a disaster for me but then with a dozen or so other eager bikers following at breakneck speed I was the instigator of the biggest mass of twisted metal the Canyon Swing area must have ever seen!

Kids either crashed into my bike or each other, they were falling this way and that. Some went straight into the tree trunks dotted around the circuit, others were unfortunate to veer left and end up hurtling down the steep embankment, into the stream, falling off and getting wet in the mêlée. Sounds of metal on metal and youngsters screaming out filled the air for seconds then a silence fell over the dingle.

This eyrie noiseless atmosphere did not last long before each rider had started to pick themselves up and examine the damage on their trusted metal steed or their own bodies. Some were in a real mess. Fortune had smiled upon me and I was not actually run over by another larger bike but I still hurt. I just had the pain and broken skin from yet another fall off my bike to contend with on my body.

Not so for others in the race. Someone had hurt his ankle so much they could not walk home without the support of their friends shoulder. Another was bleeding from a deep cut on their leg. Many suffered head bumps and bruises. It was not a good day for the bikes either. I encountered a puncture. Alan came of far worse; he had twisted his handlebars and buckled his front wheel. About half of the others could only walk their cycles home that day, so great was the damage.

I was not the target of blame by the group because I fell first. It must have been a subconscious realisation that we had all pushed the boundaries of safety and skill too far as a group and we all had to suffer the consequences.

It is said somewhere that we can learn to be clever from a book but we can only learn wisdom from the experiences we have in life, especially those that go wrong. A small group of young lads learnt some wisdom that day that hopefully they would not forget.

Needless to say Alan got it in the neck from Mother having damaged his bike. He was a paperboy at the time and he had to save hard with his money to get the bike repaired. I eventually had a puncture repair kit bought and regained my mobility after a quick repair.

Others were not so lucky and tales were told between us for many a month later about the crash and its differing consequences back at home for each and every rider. One or two must have been grounded for a while as we all went quiet on the streets immediately following the escapade.

31

Burning the Field

Those long hot summers I had as a child were a treat for me but on one occasion I had made it slightly hotter than it should have been.

Along the East Lancs Road, just before the path to Wardley woods, was an old farm surrounded by its fields. The farm was not in full use by then and some of the fields had gone fallow. They were full of old corn and grasses, scorched yellow by the summer heat.

I had an affinity in those days for fire. We were brought up on coal fires and everybody knew how to lay, tend and then clean a fire from an early age. In fact as youngsters at school we regularly made match holders in Art to take home and later at secondary school metalwork pokers to tend to the fire with and toasting forks for turning bread golden brown over the coals.

Burning the Field

I used to love poking our coal fire and reading the pictures in the flames. I could see mountains or seas moving around in the heat. Some folks used to say they could read the future in the flames. Unfortunately I was more of a pyromaniac than fortune teller.

I enjoyed getting up early to make the fire in winter. Later in the day I would wrap potatoes or apples, if we had any, in tin foil, cook them in the embers and eat them whilst hot. Toast was another open fire meal readily made. Fire would fascinate me and I was a beggar for stealing or buying matches for my playing out and lighting a campfire in the woods when fantasising.

This particular day, if you have not already guessed, I was intent on making a fire next to the woods in the farmer's field. There I was with the small crew from the Drive, Ken, Mitch and I. Gathering the grass was easy and I soon sparked them into life. Up the flames went, fanned by the dry breeze and sparks flew straight into the adjoining field.

The dry grass quickly caught fire and we all panicked as it rapidly caught hold. We tried to dowse the flames with our clothes. How could three little boys stop nature's worst master with just small summer jackets? Try as we might the sound and sight of the growing blaze sent fear into us all. It was an impossible task to try to stop it in its wake across the wide dry field.

We decided to scarper and leg it as fast as we could back home to the relative safety of Stonegate Drive, leaving the blaze to do its worst. We cycled back along the cycle path as fast as our legs could peddle not passing a word between us.

In the distance we heard the clanging of the Fire Engine's bell. Someone had spotted the blaze and rang 999 for fire brigade support. We stopped and stared as we were making our way, away from the damage and here were the rescuers making their way as fast as they could towards the danger to put the blaze out.

We stopped in someone's front garden trying to hide and prevent us from being spotted. It did not ease our panic and we just peddled off in the opposite direction of our destructive play as soon as the red engines had passed.

There could not have been any major damage or life threatening injuries because we did not read about it in the following week's local Journal paper. Mother did not find out about it and the others kept as quite about it as I did.

Even normal families would have handed of some form of corporal punishment to their children when dealing with an incident as serious as this. Good reason not to offer up an admission of guilt. Still that was a close call and I reigned in on my early pyromaniac behaviour from that day on.

32

My Sister Margaret and Our Code

Although described as a sickly child in my youth I was occasionally subject to staying off school at Mother's behest rather than any illness. You will know by now that I was often subject to a beating and well, some day's Mother had gone too far and I think she knew it.

There were nights the nagging would go on for hours. I would be stood in the cold hall, in the corner by the door so she could sit on the bottom step opposite me much more able to carry out her venting for longer periods. I would be incredibly tired, standing there, sometimes semi clothed, taking the verbal and physical abuse for hours. Occasionally pleading for mercy and confessing to never do whatever it was ever again. This was a regular occurrence.

Sometimes we were subject to it for only an hour or so. On one occasion when Alan had not got ready properly for his Grammar School so she stripped him off and threw him outside into the front hall, naked. That only lasted for about half an hour but the trauma for Alan of being there with no clothes on must have embedded itself in him for a lifetime.

Occasionally the nagging would go on into the small hours of the morning, being shouted at and abuse thrown at me, spasmodically getting very angry and lashing out with her hand or belt. The neighbours must have heard the row through the thin glass panels in the front door. Heard but no action taken, it just was not the 'done' thing in those days.

The volume and intensity of punishment was possibly dependent upon her classification of how serious the crime had been. Often her anger was such that she would use her belt against my frail body in a continual reign of blows. The buckle end was used for extreme cases of misdemeanour such as getting up late for school or talking in bed or even breaking a pot when washing up and not telling her about it out of fear of the consequences.

The buckle hurt and often broke my skin, giving me a small bleed and leaving a red and black mark on my back, leg or arm. Mother must have seen the damage she caused whilst lashing out her punishment. As she finished her correction she sometimes made the mental decision not to let me go to school the next day especially if there was a PE lesson due.

Marks and cuts like these would have raised questions even in those Dickensian like days. She couldn't have wanted the school authorities to see the results of her handiwork and I was promptly informed the next morning that I was not being allowed to school as a punishment for my wrong doings. I can remember having to stay in bed and look at my comic books only getting up to ask if I could go to the toilet. She would occasionally shout up that she was going out to the shop. I was informed that I had to stay in bed and if she caught me out of my room I would get it when she returned. Hers was a reign of terror that stayed with me even when she was not around in the immediate vicinity.

In times like these I had one real human friend in the house, in fact at times the only one in the world, who loved me and constantly showed me kindness. It was my younger sister Margaret. She would, whenever she could, come to see me when the coast was clear after a beating and give me some crumbs of comfort.

Margret had one great advantage over my little friends in that she was real and actually lived through and heard some of the punishments herself. She said kind words about me that made me realise I had someone on this earth who knew how I felt and it was all not really my fault. She even invented a way of informing or warning me if I was to be the subject of another attack.

Mother would let the others know in the house that she had discovered something I had done wrong and then told them I was in for it when I arrived back from where ever I was. Margaret would wait upstairs in her room for ages looking out of the window for me arriving home.

When she did see me she would gain my attention and then either have her thumb up or down dependent upon mother's mood. A thumb at a right angle meant that mother was not in a good mood but it was nothing specific or directed at me in particular. A thumb down meant that I was to incur the wrath of another session. I at least was ready and knew that after it was all over Margaret would wait for me and then offer her comfort to me.

What she really felt when I was on the receiving end I have not had the courage to ask her, even today. I wonder if she had the foresight to know she pulled me through some very bad days that had sometimes made me think of a permanent exit from the situation I found myself trapped in.

She was my human angel sent to maintain my sanity and give me a hope that it would all end one day. We all must look for our angels that are sent to us. They are there; sometimes we just do not look hard enough or choose to ignore them when they appear.

My wife, Rachel, is my angel of today. She has given me the courage to uncover myself after nearly a full lifetime of being unable to unlock the past, let it go, thus enabling me to clear my way for the future.

Find your angel and offer them back the love and kindness they give you, only tenfold. Margaret was my first angel and our bond and love for each other is as strong today as it was then, even if we do have to send it over the miles to Toronto where she now lives.

33

Rape!

Although summer was my favourite time for playing out one hot day, did hold a particular difficult and viciously painful time for me. This was the one occasion that mother was not involved or the cause of such physical pain and mental trauma that I had to endure.

It was a typical long sunny day; I would still have been at junior school, about nine or ten. Swinton was not as rough as the centre of Salford but it still had more than its fair share of rouges and villains. This day I met two evil people who hurt me in a way even I had never been damaged before or ever want to again.

I have mentioned the wonderland of adventure called the Clough, filled with steep gullies, streams and small wild life. I would cycle down there on my old Phillips bike with its steel wired brakes, bottle of water and slices of bread in a bag slung from its rusty handlebars. Losing myself in activity, play and my fantasies, I could change the course of the streams with dams and construction work using only the natural materials found there. I also was forever hiding in the small undergrowth playing war games by myself, pretending to conquer evil or being a super animal surviving in jungle conditions. Mother and her cruel regime could have been a million miles away.

This particular day the fantasy world I created crashed into reality with an evil stroke of misfortune. I happened to be in the wrong place at the wrong time. A trick I have unwittingly mastered and fell foul of all my life although not necessarily with such damaging effects as this particular day.

I was building up of the many stream diverting mud, stick and stone creations when I was shouted at from the top of the gully. This gully was a part where the stream could not easily be seen from the path along the top or the main road at the end before it disappeared into the concrete tunnel taking it under the East Lancashire Road.

A good haven for me to play undisturbed, yet this secret place contributed to my attack. "Hey you, Ginger, have you got any money?" Looking up I saw two boys, about five or six years older than I was, clambering down the dry mud embankment towards me.

"Money?" I thought, "I never have any!"

"No," I meekly answered knowing these two were capable of giving me much trouble "I have not got any, just a bottle of water,"

Rape!

They were both much bigger than me and the nearest one was big enough to be working. He had a faint beard, bum fluff we called it, as if he had never shaved trying to grow an 'adult' impression. It gave him a dirty look, unkempt and unwashed.

"I bet you have," was his reply as he rushed down the embankment towards me. He promptly put his hands into my trouser pockets to search for any coins. His mate stood next to him and looked around as if on the lookout for witnesses. I knew I was in for some bad treatment. I instantly felt the fear I regularly had at home when Mother collared me and was about to launch into one of her violent attacks on my body.

I mentioned before the summer Khaki pants I wore were hard wearing but they did have an Achilles heel. The two front pockets were made from ordinary cotton and soon wore holes in them from my over carrying of items like stones, an assortment of toys and little tools.

This big lad placed his hand into my pockets and his fingers went straight on to my genital area. He held one of my testicles with his hand and squeezed hard. I cried out with the pain and shock but his grip was so tight I could not move away and break his strangle hold.

"No money ginger," he mocked, "Well I will just have to have these instead." He placed his other hand in my left pocket, grabbed my left testicle. I remember him fondling my penis and testicles then his attitude changed and became more menacing. From behind he pushed his groin against my backside and squeezed my body in a lock that took my breath away.

My mind was confused, what's he doing? Why do I feel so frightened? I remember most of his actions vividly. He stunk of cigarette smoke and a staleness I sometimes re-smell when I walk past someone who has not washed on a regular basis. It is a smell that haunts me today whenever I catch it. I could not describe him or his mate's physical features but that smell lingers inside my subconscious inner self.

"Watch out," he told his mate who promptly turned on his heels and looked around. At this I remember him picking me up by forcing his arms in a bear hug against my smaller body and lifting. I felt faint from the pressure he exerted on my stomach and chest.

He started carrying me towards a large overgrown shrub I knew had a den inside it. I tried to kick his shin with the back of my foot but he just tightened his grip on me. I stilled and felt limp. What was he going to do, give me a good hammering for not having any money for him? I was soon to find out and the reality of my plight was to be worse, so bad it has taken nearly 50 years for me to retell. Retell it I must for the nightmares I still have linger on.

He stood me up and turned me around towards him. I remember him shouting out to his accomplice to let him know if anyone comes in sight. His face was only inches away from mine as his hands went to the five buttons that fastened my shorts. He kept smiling as he softly said "We'll see if you have anything for me Ginger." Quickly he pulled my pants and underpants down then played with my penis for a short while.

I was so afraid. I could not shout or scream. I just recall it all as if in slow motion and in a silence like the films when they want to emphasise a particularly horrific part of the film.

He turned my body away from him and pushed me to the ground, face down. I felt a sharp pain in my groin as he prised my legs as far apart as they would go. The muscles in my legs hurt, that sharp pain similar to cramp but much more acute. He hit the back of my head hard with a stick. That I remember because the stick broke and it fell in pieces next to my face. Then he entered me.

I cannot remember if I screamed out loud or if it was in my head. It was a sharp stabbing pain I felt. Today just on occasions I feel it again when I strain going to the toilet. I just lay there, his weight making my breathing difficult and I was choking on my tears and the dirt I was in pushed into went into my mouth. A very strange feeling for me, I could feel his penis pulsating inside me. It was not painful as his initial entrance had been. I just cried. His warm sperm made the nerves around my anus tingle.

My emotions were all over the place and my thoughts were in disarray. It felt like a flood. I sobbed uncontrollably coughing and spluttering on the dirt. His mate soon appeared in the hidden space inside the bush. It was his turn for the prize. I suffered less when he repeated the rape. I must have been in shock for I recall the initial searing pain but not the second time yet it must have hurt as badly.

The bigger bully gave his parting words "Tell anyone and well come back and kill you." I really thought at the time he meant it; people like him were a law unto themselves and would do whatever they said they would. I never knew such fear outside of my house. I had never seen them ever before that day and never saw them again. Yet their fifteen or so minutes of fun still disturb my sleep.

When I dream about it, it makes me wake at three or four in the morning and stay wide awake till the dawn brings light to my sad situation. Where was my God in all this, you might wonder. Well I can only suggest he saw and cried along with me, feeling my pain.

I never felt anger towards the two evil people or the need for retribution. Perhaps God gave me a glimmer of His gentleness when I recall the act. The only feelings I have for those two is that they must have been in great need of repair inwardly. Perhaps knowing my God in the way I do would have helped them, who knows?

I have two reoccurring dreams around my rape. One is where I am still on the spot where it happened. I have an old fashioned foot pump inserted into my anus. It is a long upright brass one with a wooden handle and two feet rests to help steady it.

Often my Mother is pumping it and I just inflate with air. Fatter and fatter I get then up and up I go floating in to the air. All the time I shout "I did not do it. It was not my fault. You never believe me." I often disappear into the great blue sky to diminish behind a cloud, never to be seen again.

Rape!

The other nightmare is more sinister. I am in a wooded area that I do not know and a large werewolf type animal attacks me from behind. It is the pet of the two boys that raped me and they are stood at the side laughing. The beast pins me down and takes its large sharp claw then slices me open from throat down to penis. All my inner organs are on show. I just lay there bleating. Sometime it eats my organs, other times it runs off when the boys call it to them. I always wake up at this point.

I dare say some dream analyst reading this will be able to unpick and analyse it all. I just want it to go away and hope that this wordy recall will help my rehabilitation. Whilst I have been writing the whole distressing episode for you I must say it has recurred. The nightmare awoke me today after spending yesterday outlining the basis of the attack on my computer.

My dearest wife Rachel has comforted me and gives me the quiet reassurance I need to carry on. Why has it taken so long to find and fall in love with her? She is the greatest therapy I could ever have or need on this earth.

Back in time and on the Clough I can unfortunately remember the trauma far too vividly. As shaken by the mental trauma as I was; as soon as they had run off I went to put my underpants and shorts back on.

Perhaps embarrassment overcame fear; shame beat the horror of the whole incident. I cried out, "ARGGGGH" as I turned over and lent towards my clothes a piercing pain sheared through my rear.

Panicking I thought that I would have to tell the

ambulance people and get treatment. No, whatever I had just been subject to had to end here. I could not continue the trauma and tell others what had gone on. I must keep it a secret, my shame was too great. They would all tell me it was my fault and I would have to pay for it. I asked for it and who is bothered about a naughty little boy anyway.

Besides, Mother will vent her anger on me yet again. I will not let her kill me for being raped, only I knew how I felt and how innocent I was. Yet I felt so guilty. What was I to do? I could not bend over to get dressed again and there was blood running down each leg. Perhaps the best thing to do would be to just lay here until I was better, and then go home.

I remember I keep crying partly because of the pain and partly because I thought I had brought it on myself. How deep the pit I must have been in, with such steep unscalable sides, that I only wanted it to collapse on top of me to end the incident and me.

The timing was such that it was early afternoon and I had plenty of time to 'get myself better' and cover up my little mishap! The three siblings, Margaret, Alan and I were never good at lying. We were always found out but there were other ways of the truth not being held against us as the kick start for any punishment.

Into the dirty stream I cupped my hand and washed away the blood from my legs. The wound must have stopped most of the bleeding now so I gently levered my underpants and khaki shorts up my legs to their rightful place. I ripped leaves from the bushes and stuffed them into my underpants. They were hard and made me sore but I was sure it helped the blood from getting noticed. My pathetic state must not be noticed by the outside world.

People would not understand because they were not there and did not see what really went on. Whatever I said I would not be believed. They would just tell me it happed a particular way and I would be blamed. That was the way it always was and just my lot in life.

I managed to slowly and gingerly clamber up the steep embankment to the path and my bike above. My anus started to give me pain again. I tried to look around to see if it was showing the blood but could not see. I felt wet so blood must have still been leaking. What could I do to get home undetected?

My little brown corduroy jacket rescued me. I placed it on my hips and tied the sleeves around the front of my waist. It was not perfect but the best ploy I could think of. Now I just needed to walk off the Clough, then the length of the road, cross Partington Lane and finally hobble home.

If anyone stops me I could say I just fell off my bike. I must have looked a real sight. Dirt all over my clothes and body, hobbling up the road pushing my old blue bike, eyes red from crying and generally dishevelled in appearance. Time was not counted, it must have been an age yet I had no recollection of how long it all took me.

Fortune smiled on me, this brave little chap, no one was around till I got to the main road. I waited for a break in the traffic then tried to run across the tarmac divide.

An arrow shot into my backside and I nearly fainted with pain. I could not run, it was too traumatic for my physically damaged area. My hobbling must have been seen by others, yet not one of the people passing stopped or interfered with my plight. I managed to get across and rested against the large red brick wall of the cobblers shop on the corner.

All my fears and thoughts began to turn to how I was to get past the stringent screening of mother. My fragile world would be broken into millions of unbearable pieces if She found out.

34

Mrs Bleasant

Up our Drive I shuffled a pathetic little snivelling wreck. Only Mrs Bleasent was out, tending her front garden, gently hoeing the weeds out between the green and yellow privet hedges. She was another lovely warm older woman in my life, my surrogate grandmother on the Drive. A slightly plump lady in her fifties, she never worked with a job but was always washing, cleaning and baking.

Hers was an open house that forever smelt of food and fresh flowers. She would invite the children into her home to eat the left over pastry from her baking or take some of the small mince pies she made continually through the year. She was yet another ultimate personification of kindness and motherliness.

The Bleasent's were also the first family on our drive to have a Television. Regularly in summer at around five o'clock the kids from the drive were invited in to watch the unveiling of the little nine inch box from under its knitted cover. We all sat in awe cross-legged on Mrs Bleasent's back room floor watching it warm up. In silence then we watched the only children's programme for the day. When it was finished we were scuttled out to play and re-enact the programme we had just indulged in.

To use the modern day vernacular it gave us such 'street cred' as we went to school to ask if our peers watched such and such programme on TV last night knowing full well only about 10% had TVs then.

This fateful day Mrs Bleasent noticed me whilst she cleared up her front garden. "Oh dear Christopher," she looked down at me, "What have you been doing?"

"I've fallen off my bike on the Clough Mrs Bleasent," came my mumbled reply.

"Well make sure your mother gets you a bath and puts a plaster on you cuts," she said in a soothing manner.

I often wondered why James Bleasent should be an only child? His parent's could have had me then I could play with the room size train set that was permanently out in their front room. I would have eaten home-made cakes every day and had a bed time story read to me with her large warm arms wrapped around me in my bed.

I could feel her huge, soft eyes watching me as I trundled up to my house and pushed the bike along the short steep path to the side. She could not have guessed the trauma I had just suffered I prayed to myself.

I was approaching my house, I had to think fast. I know,

I would put the bike around the back of the coal shed then go and hide in the shed for a while. As I passed the kitchen window mother caught a glimpse of my ginger mop. "Are you coming in for your tea?" she asked. Her sentence finished in a long cough. It gave me time to think of a good answer.

"I'm going to put my bike away then wash. I fell off my bike and got dirt all over me."

"You had better not have ripped your clothes," she kept coughing as she spoke. "I can't afford new clothes and your next lot are for school when you go back," she emphasised the 'I' giving the sentence a slant towards her personal plight.

The effort of trying to talk whilst ridding her air sacks of the foul covering of tar was too much and she went into the back room to sit and 'cough her lungs up'. Often she did this and then spat the phlegm into a ripped off piece of the Manchester Evening News before depositing it in the fire place. No fire on such a warm summer day as today but she could still transfer it into a sheet of the evening paper to rid herself of the tacky dark mixture.

I froze as I went around the back of the coal shed. Was the French window open and could she see me from behind? Luckily for me it was not and I could hear her coughing from behind the thin glass and metal frame. This attack enabled me to slide past the open door to the back room and get up stairs to the bathroom.

Bearing in mind the hot water was only ever put on when we were having visits from her sisters I washed with tepid water from the hot tap. Pulling my underpants down I felt the dried blood sticking to my skin and deciding whether to peel off the clothes or let them remain attached to me.

I could only look in disbelief as I saw inside of my shorts. They were covered in blood. What was I to do with them? I let them fall onto the lino and I cleaned up my skin from the effects of the attack with a flannel. I did not dare approach my anus with the soap and water; it was far too tender and raw. I dried my legs then put my ear next to the door of the bathroom. I could only hear mother downstairs clattering around the kitchen.

Now was my chance, bundling my tell tale clothing under my arm I crept out of the stark bathroom into my bedroom. I pulled clean shorts over my dirty underpants making sure I opened the draw of my chest slowly and silently. This was lest the owl like ears of her downstairs heard and came running up to burst open the door and shout "What the hell do you need to go into your draws for at this time of the day?"

I hid my clothes of guilt underneath the bottom draw. It was a secret place where I could keep items I did not want mother to find. Alan and Margaret were not around and I had time to think. I had to destroy these reminders of my fate, sexual abuse victims always feel dirty after being attacked and I needed to cleanse myself. Washing my skin again and again and then destroying the soiled clothing was the only option. I washed and washed myself in the cold tap water several times later that day and for many days after.

My clothes were a different matter. I was to take out them later in the week when I was alone at home and I buried them in the soil on the Indoo's, far away from the spot where I was attacked. It was the only place I could think of where Mother would never find the evidence. I slept with two pairs of underpants and pyjama bottoms on that night.

Long before Alan came up to bed I lay there, recalling in my head the ordeal and feeling that I was such a low life. Yet again in my sad life I just wanted to die. Never in my times of punishment and beatings from Mother had I felt such a hurt as this one. I was so hollow, ashamed and dirty, a victim of my own evil, I thought.

God, why did you let it happen? Where were you when I needed you to come down and strike those two dead? You saw it; I know you did, why oh why did you let it happen to me? Did you think I deserved it? Why did I not have a dad who was here and could go find the evil thugs and beat the living daylights out of them? These were the instant thoughts my mind wrestled with.

But I knew that God had been there and later, much later I was being told another story from the Good Book about forgiveness that I started to think about my perpetrators. Could I forgive them as Jesus forgave those who persecuted him to His death? "Father, forgive them," He asked as they killed Him mercilessly, "For they know not what they do."

Was I really big enough inside my soul to say to them in my head "Sorry," not for me, but for them? Having God in your life never makes things easier; He just lets you know what you should do in very difficult situations. Often it is as difficult to deal with in His way but always just and right.

Needless to say I was very quiet for a while and did not venture to the Clough to play the rest of that holiday. My head was traumatised with inner fighting on the act for many hours, days and weeks to come. I gradually and slowly let its psychological pain go, buried into the back of my inner self, only to resurface when such incidents of cruelty and torture are brought into the public domain by others and opinions are aired or requested.

They still can today, I can't put into words here just how difficult it has been to write these last chapters even today so far away from the event and go over them again to check my spelling or grammar. The wound may have healed, but the scar is still there as a permanent reminder.

35

My Swan Song
at Moorside School

The final chapter of my early life comes just before the transition from the juniors to senior school at the age of eleven. It was a transition that I recall with some humour, a little pride and a sense of growing up and having found some direction to aim for in my life.

Before that final Christmas in the juniors each of the three fourth year classes were told that we could have a concert and all the pupils could perform in front of the rest of the school. The front of the hall was to be our stage and we could use the record player that amplified into speakers if we needed.

That put a real buzz amongst those who were departing Moorside that year. We could perform a swan song before leaving to the senior schools that was to be of our educational home for the next four or five years.

Around the January or February all the last year pupils took the 11 plus grading test and we had worked hard towards it since September. The concert should be some light relief for all.

In 4W, my middle set, I was party to being friends with small group of likely lads; James Carpenter and Sandy Daniels were just two of the bunch. I hasten to say I was also brushed with the same colour paint by the staff although I always thought myself as different, better in fact than the other two.

To be classed as part of the gang you had to have a fight with at least two of the others to determine your rank in the group. I had mine with Sandy and got soundly beaten. He was classed as the 'hardest' in the school! I was on to a looser before it began but it gave me the recognition I needed to become a part and not picked on as an outsider.

Sandy was the real villain of the piece at Moorside, he, even as a young eleven year old would bunk off school every Friday afternoon to ride his older brother's motor cross motorbike in the woods. Who else would get away with that at such a tender age?

He showed me how to go into a shop and nick sweets from the counter, setting up a decoy by someone else buying, dithering with their purchase. This distracted the shopkeeper so he could help himself to treats he shared amongst us later. This was an insight to his wayward life as a real 'handful' and he grew into a large beast of a man.

James Carpenter was different, a likable rogue, more cheeky than evil with who I had an altercation earlier in my school life. This conflict did give us a bond as we grew up together in the educational system. I had nicked his balaclava one day from his peg in the cloak room and went home with it on. His mother went ballistic and caused a stink back at school. Guess who had to own up to the evil deed, little old me?

Mother near killed me back at home, not for the crime but her embarrassment at having to face the other mothers after her son was deemed a thief. Well the balaclava was better than mine and I needed a new one, why could I not recycle it, James could easily get another one, they lived in a nice house! That train of thought had no resilience in Mother's eyes. I never stole another balaclava after that, believe me, lesson leant!

Or maybe it was more a case of fear of the punishment greater than the benefits of gaining a new item of clothing. I had to stand in the hall being nagged for hours that day with the occasional slapping of the belt to keep me awake. Needless to say I was not allowed to return to school for at least 24 hours, till the marks had gone.

The preparations for this Christmas concert were actually held in the classroom each week. The teacher would have a set amount of marking to do and would normally set us work, to keep us quiet, whilst she sat at her high desk and ticked or otherwise the outcomes from her learners. What she did do was a free thinking, spontaneous act of genius unheard of in such a rigid educational establishment.

She turned over that time to us to organise ourselves to practice performing at the front before the others in the room. James, Sandy and I held a brief meeting over Sandy's desk and we came to the conclusion that this school needed a good dose of new music. The Beatles were our answer, a new young, up and coming group who kicked the teeth of the establishment. "Let's sing some Beatles numbers and shock the school." Wow, the idea was awesome and I immediately called upon my vast repertoire of musical talent and chipped in. "Can I be Ringo cos I can play the drums?"

"Yea," Sandy replied "And I'm John Lennon." This left James with a choice Paul or George.

"I'll be the other two," was the answer to the difficulty and from that moment on a slice of musical history in Moorside was born.

One girl in the class wanted to recite a poem, how boring I thought, just like school lessons. Other pupils brought records in to sing to, one did a Cilla Black song. Cilla was all the rage at the time but the miming left us three cold. We were real and I was determined to make this a concert the kids and staff would remember for years to come.

We started to write down the words to songs such as 'Twist and Shout' to the best of our ability for our intro song. James could get hold of a guitar. It was a Spanish one and made of polished wood but it had a strap on to go over your shoulder and I said we could tie string onto it to make it look like an electric one. Sandy also managed to get his hands on a guitar, where from we never asked! That just left me to make the most of impersonating Ringo. I had one military side drum at home from the Church Lads

Brigade so that had to be a part of the kit. I managed to scrounge one tin biscuit box and a large pan from the kitchens. With my best drum sticks I was complete!

I always regarded the kitchen ladies at Moorside as my friends; they smiled on me and always repaid my friendliness at 'seconds' time. I would chat to them as if they were aunties and I helped them enormously every day with their washing up. Not by doing the job, you must understand, and getting my hands wet but helping to clear their enormous aluminium cooking pots of custard skin.

To get your dinner in the hall at lunch time we all had to queue in silence with a plate as the domiciliary staff dished out the fruits of their morning labours from their hatches. When it came to puddings it would always be rhubarb and custard or spotted dick and custard or even apple crumble and custard.

The yellow sweet was made in such large dishes that they always had a thick skin across the top. This was carefully pulled aside revealing the movable liquid inside that could be dished out and slid around the dish. When it came to 'seconds', food left over after everyone had been fed, I was always up for trying to fill my belly as compensation for the mean meals we endured at home.

For some reason, which I could never understand, this thick edible belly filler called custard skin was never acceptable food to the other kids I went to school with. Not me, I revelled in it and would walk on my own with my plate to the large dishes and offer the empty dish up, Oliver style. Then the kind old lass on the other side of the counter would fill to the brim my dish with this unwanted food source.

'Seconds' ensured my meal intake at school compensated for the lack of a balanced, healthy quantity of food I endured under the miserly regime at home. The kitchen ladies actually played their part in my call to emulate the stars of the day.

Our dynamic trio talked continually at play times in the yard and would plan and plot every aspect, even sang Beatles' songs to get the right vibes and remember the words. I say sang, singing was not our strongest aspect as a group. 'Front' was! We felt a mile high, buzzing with anticipation and could not wait for the day when we 'hit' the other kids with our little show.

Dress sense was compiled from whatever we could get our hands on. I had a pair of bronze jeans that my brother had previously bought from his earning as a paper boy and sadly for him, grown out of. They were really hip, cool and trendy for their day with a real turn up. I also had a leather sleeveless waistcoat that I previously used in a dance performance which would take its part.

Sadly for me the Beatles had mops of shaggy hair which I struggled to emulate. All I had was just a curly ginger haired covering that was cut short, as deemed as the tradition for boys in its day. It was incredibly important to get a mop, as their hair was their single most important trademark that defined them visually. Unfortunately,this was definitely the era of short back and sides or square necks for all the men and boys, a standard scoffed at by the Fab Four.

Then the idea of the year hit me! I could use a domestic mop head as my hair and I would be the most original Beatle Moorside had ever seen. Back to my friendly neighbourhood dinner ladies I trotted and offered my request hoping against hope that they saw the imagination behind my idea and gave me their blessing (and spare mop head). Amid the chuckles from the ladies an old dirty fluffy cloth head appeared. They did relinquish it to me under a sworn request that they could watch me perform in the show and I was to let them know when it was.

This was bread and butter to me, a receptive audience that had a positive stake in my antics. I told mother next to nothing at home, managing to take the drum out of the house by saying I was playing it as part of a concert. To become a Beatle would be taboo to her; the adult public had not yet taken on board the musical skills and enormity of those four scouse lads. They were too often seen in the early days as just long haired trouble makers from Liverpool, of all places. Mother would definitely not have approved.

The great day came and the programme said we were to go on the stage last. I say stage, imagine a large parquet floored hall with the doors to the corridor at one end and an area in front of the gym mats and ropes where the teachers stood in assemblies facing the rest of the school. The acoustics were not ideal, no stage lighting or even a raised platform but we were in our element.

The performance began and various kids filed forward to

perform their 'entertainment' for the rest of the school. We followed the little girl singer who mimed to Cilla Black and she was politely clapped by the rest of the pupils.

Then we arrived. I took two chairs, turned them to face me and placed them next to each other at the back of our performance area. Positioning the drum then pan and biscuit tin I nodded to my two other 'musicians' that I was almost ready. I then ran back to the side where I had placed the mop head.

In practice it just would not stay onto my head so after another brainwave I had asked for a length of sticky back plastic from the office and stuck it right across the mop with enough length to go under my chin. It went straight on to my ginger nut and I pulled the tape around and under my chin. It worked, nodding a few times to trial its stability the old mop stuck on and I was ready to hit the school big time.

I rushed back on with a drumstick in each hand and the crowd of kids started to laugh and roar at me. Music to my ears, it was sweet success, a whole junior school laughing with me and not at me and we had not started to perform. This instantly gave me the 'power of the performance' which filled me with confidence and I knew I could perform my utmost for the crowd.

Sandy struck up singing the first number, 'Love me do' and we rocked the joint. All the little seven to eleven year olds who were use to conforming to the establishment when in the hall clapped and sang spontaneously and at the top of their voices. It was like a rebellion for us all and I, yes

I was playing a lead part in it. I bashed away in time, having a sense of rhythm which by then covered the inadequacies of me not being able to drum a set of skins. My pleasure was exhibited by my writhing around and dancing to the song whilst beating the tins. I must have looked a sight but felt so cool. We ended the first song to rousing applause.

The teaching staff who were stood along the sides of the hall to 'police' the concert were laughing loudly and clapping along with the rest of the children. I loved it! This was my homecoming in a school that for so many years had been my place of torture, ridicule and hell. I felt I was king. So much for all the canings and beatings I had, this was the real me and I was loving it.

Sandy turned round and said, "Please please me OK?" I was off, confidence sky high and shouted whilst beating the time so professionally,

"One two, a one two three four!" Fortunately Sandy and James followed and burst into song. My antics with the sticks grew and when it came to the lines 'If there's anything that you want',I shouted at a volume reserved only for watching the rugby matches at Swinton, "Fish and Chips!"

Totally unrehearsed this should have thrown the two singers completely off course but they just carried on in time. "If there's anything I can do?"

"Pass the salt!" was my reply. The hall was in hysterics. I had caused belly laughs with all my peers and with the staff. It was the greatest feeling I had ever experienced in school and possibly was ever likely to.

I rocked, danced and pranced through the song and at the end the crowd went wild. They stood up (absolutely unheard of at Moorside) and clapped and cheered at the three Beatles that had broken taboos and entertained, yes entertained staff children and a line of laughter filled tearful dinner ladies stood at the back.

My ego had never been in this uncharted territory before and I realised that I had a skill to make people happy, laugh and like me, yes actually like me. That day I realised there was a power the stage gave me right across the board with people of all ages. It was the beginning of a step into small time fame that was to keep me entertaining people right up to today in one guise or another. A star was born, no matter how dimly lit it shone, and it was me.

From that day onwards those blessed dinner ladies always made sure my plate was piled high whenever I was in the queue for lunch. I remain eternally grateful for them having the faith in me to carry out the transformation into a pop star with the aid of their floor cleaning implement, the humble mop head!

36

That Damned
Eleven Plus Exam

There was, in those days, a previously mentioned streaming process based upon academic ability. The greatest turning point in the last year on juniors came when all pupils sat the national exam called the Eleven-plus. It was an IQ test meant to siphon off the clever kids into Grammar schools so they could be educated with their peers in academic subjects and eventually go to Higher Education.

This small percentage of genius was expected to fill the Universities when leaving school at eighteen after their 'A' level exams. Those who failed the eleven-plus at such an early age were left to learn more practical subjects like woodwork and cooking. Little was expected from them and they offered little themselves.

It was usual that they left school at fifteen to gain an

apprenticeship or at sixteen after taking their 'O' level exams. It was a great directional point in a young child's life and the consequences of missing this bus into a Grammar school could be grave, especially for their parents!

I was naturally expected to become a member of the latter, less educated group and be assigned to it by failing my eleven-plus. Little did my teachers or family realise my full potential. I bucked the suggested trend and passed!

The letter that said I had been successful came and was able to go to Salford Technical High, my first choice of selected secondary school. Mother would like to think it was because of the workbooks she bought me prior to the exam and made me sit through working away at. I like to think it was because of it being more of an IQ test and my IQ was such that it was greater than the masking of dyslexia had proved. Unfortunately again for me, Moorside offered one final swipe at my curse in the short time before I left.

The headmaster was a very quiet man who never journeyed into the classroom but spent his time locked in the vast chair he had in his office shuffling paper around on his desk. A short very rounded bald man he always wore tweeds and had a musty smell about him. He nonchalantly dawdled into school with his short sausage dog trotting behind, briefcase in one hand and cushion for his dog in the other.

I only visited him when I was being caned for some humongous crime that rocked the educational establishment such as using a swearword or being sent out of class on more than three occasions in a week. Neither did my mother have any dealings with him.

In those days parents were left at the gates of educational premises, inside it was the educational staff that had sole responsibility and contact with the children. I remember he made a special event of seeing my mother after I had passed my exam. I was not privy to the conversation but mother relayed it to me as such. "Your headmaster said he was surprised that you had passed the eleven-plus but said he wished me well and also said you would be better off in a Technical High school instead of a Grammar school, where I would find it difficult to concentrate and keep up with the work, not being that clever."

A fitting misguided tribute to a pupil who had, against all odds, at home and at school, survived the system and managed to throw a final statement of high intellect into the ring by passing such a hard external exam. Little did he know the difficulties and adventures I was to have on the next ladder in life that I was about to climb? How false and true at the same time were his words to be.

The next chapter of my troubled journey was about to begin or, more accurately, I was ready to stumble into adolescent action.

Beth Moulam

Beth Moulam is a young lady with very profound Cerebral Palsy and no voice of her own. She speaks through a communication machine and leads training sessions for staff and others based around her life skills and positive attitude.

Beth was twelve when I first met her and her words helped me to face my fears. The quotes I have used of hers are taken from her life story, so inspiring to listen to.

She is a fantastic role model for me and many others, especially younger people. She has qualities that I wish I had at her age, then I know I could have coped with my difficulties far better.

People in this world need other people like Beth to set them good examples of how to live life to the full without hurting others or taking away from them. A real positive role model, thanks Beth, you have certainly inspired me.